Be Your Own
Makeup Artist

Be Your Own Makeup Artist

JEROME ALEXANDER'S Complete Makeup Workbook

by
JEROME ALEXANDER
and
ROBERTA ELINS

HARPER & ROW, PUBLISHERS, New York
Cambridge, Philadelphia, San Francisco, London
Mexico City, São Paulo, Sydney
1817

Photography: Patrice Casanova
Illustrations and Art Direction: Alan M. Biller
Art Production: Stacy Antokas
Hair (book jacket): Eisaburo Ishikawa of Yves Claude Hair
All makeup: Jerome Alexander

FIRST EDITION

Designer: Abigail Sturges

Library of Congress Cataloging in Publication Data

Alexander, Jerome.
  Be your own makeup artist.

  Includes index.
  1. Beauty, Personal.   2. Cosmetics.   I. Elins, Roberta.   II. Title.
RA778.A437   1983   646.7′26   82–48107
ISBN 0–06–015088–2

83 84 85 86 87   10 9 8 7   6 5 4 3 2 1

To my wife, Geraldine, who is beauty personified and who has given me our wonderful son, Berin. Merely being around her is an inspiration to all things beautiful.

To my dearest friend, Larry Mathews, who started me in the beauty business, has always given me his total support, and has remained my closest confidant.

—Jerome Alexander

To my husband, Gary Hitzig, whose constant love and support always make me feel beautiful.

To my mother, Florence Schoenbrun, whose unique love has given me the freedom to be me.

—Roberta Elins

Contents

Introduction

For twenty-five years I have been involved in teaching women how they can look their most beautiful. I've made up the top models, the celebrities, and have given advice to visiting dignitaries. But that is not the source of my strength. I believe that my contribution has been "keeping America (and the rest of the world) beautiful." Women from New York to California and every point in between, as well as the women of Paris, Milan, and London, have learned to be a little more beautiful with my help.

My career as beauty maker started as an odd job to continue my education. While putting myself through school, I sold cosmetics to women at house parties. But instead of just hawking creams and powders in a variety of colors, I showed these women *how to apply cosmetics* for maximum results. I experienced the excitement a woman feels when she sees herself become more beautiful.

The businessman in me saw the volume of my sales grow. Women didn't want just to buy cosmetics; they wanted fulfillment of the promise cosmetics offer—to look more beautiful. They wanted a beauty education; I became the educator. Selling makeup had been a means to an end, but somewhere, at one of those selling parties, the makeup artist in me was born, and the means became the end. I was in the beauty business.

My first significant contribution to the world of beauty came during the 1960s with my wig business. The sixties was the decade of flips, falls, and curly mops. Women saw wigs as the liberators of limp, thin, and unmanageable hair. I saw wigs for what they were: heavy, uncomfortable, poorly designed, and, most of all artificial-looking. I successfully set out to change the conception of wigs. If women wanted to change their image through wigs—if they wanted to have fun with hair—I believed they should be able to do it with quality and style.

Jerome Alexander Wigs became the designer name in the wig industry. No longer were wigs a bargain-basement item but designer signatures for the head. By the time the craze for wigs started to wane, the Jerome Alexander name was the haute couture of wigs.

The love affair women had with wigs never developed into a long-term relationship, and the seventies saw me return to my first love—cosmetics. In 1976, Jerome Alexander Cosmetics was born. The cosmetics industry is indisputably one of the toughest in the world. There is very little room for a new kid on the block. But the giants of the industry didn't know women the way I did.

Those early years of crisscrossing the country, talking to women, listening to women, and teaching them paid off. I knew what the beauty-conscious woman was missing in her cosmetics wardrobe—the tools that are the mainstay of every makeup artist and every successful model. Women were buying expensive blushers, eye shadows, and lipsticks that came with dime-store, toylike applicators. They were frustrated and confused when they couldn't duplicate the results cosmetic advertisements promised.

I wasn't confused. I knew that for the proper results, the right tools were essential. I put the tools of the professional into the hands of the consumer. Quality brushes, applicators, and sponge wedges, once found only in the makeup artist's toolbox, were now on bureaus and in handbags all over the world. And because I never sold a woman a product without educating her in its use, a "how-to" booklet instructing women in the proper use of tools was included in every brush kit. I didn't just want to sell products; I wanted to sell beauty—and that meant continuing my role as an educator.

Jerome Alexander Cosmetics was a success from its inception. In addition to my knowledge of what women want, I filled a unique niche in the cosmetic world. Though there were many beauty queens, now there was a man educating women in the art of being beautiful.

Today, my company is known for innovative colors, products, and quality tools. I have not stopped being the professor of beauty. Grueling cross-country trips to reach the women of America are still part of my yearly itinerary. Women are still learning from me, and I *never* stop learning from them.

Now, in this book, I'm going to reveal all the secrets of the professional makeup artist. Twenty-five years of experience, tips, tricks, and illusions are going to be in your hands.

John Cage once wrote: "Where does beauty begin and where does it end? Where it ends is where the artist begins." I will teach you to become your own makeup artist.

Acknowledgments

We would like to thank the following people for contributing their unique talents to *Be Your Own Makeup Artist:* Helen Moore, editor; Helen Barrett and Pam Bernstein, literary agents; Patrice Casanova, photographer; Alan Biller, illustrator and art director; Stacy Antokas, art production; Eisaburo Ishikawa, hair stylist; Peggy Messina and Marianne Milligan, researchers; Annick Berns, manuscript typist.

In addition, we would like to thank the following people for their invaluable support and direction from the time the book was just an idea: Robert Feldman, Suzee Kornfeld, Carole Bidnick, Robert Knight, and Christopher Ward.

Be Your Own Makeup Artist

1. Brushes and Tools

Brushes. Sponges. Applicators. Puffs. Tools. Implements. Find a professional makeup artist and you'll find as many tools and brushes as you will find cosmetics. Whether the professional is doing a theatrical makeup, makeup for movies or television, fashion makeup, or an everyday makeup, he or she knows that *without the right tools it is virtually impossible* to achieve professional-looking results.

Today, more attention is being given to the importance of professional brushes and tools for the application of makeup, and the availability of brushes and tools to the consumer is becoming more widespread. I remember when obtaining the proper tools was not an easy task—not even for the professional make-up artist.

When I first started doing makeup in the late 1950s, I literally had to create my own brushes. I would go to an artist's supply store and buy the finest brushes available. The thinnest artist's brush, which I would purchase to use as a fine eyeliner brush, was still too thick to properly apply eyeliner. So, using a razor, I would shape the brushes until they were adaptable to cosmetics. Fashioning my own brushes was time-consuming and expensive. I might ruin five sable brushes before I had a brush that would work the way I wanted it to.

Sponge-foam wedges, which are invaluable to a makeup artist for blending and applying color, were also a self-made tool. I would have to order foam from an upholstery supplier and cut it into inch-thick triangles.

Eventually, brushes began to be available to professional makeup artists at some professional outlets, mainly theatrical makeup suppliers. Life was a little easier for the professional artist, but the consumer was still left with inefficient, inexpensive applicators that came with the product.

The realization that something had to be done about this situation came to me in 1976 when I was walking through a department store and stopped to watch a makeup artist do a makeup on a customer. He used all his professional brushes and tools to apply the makeup, and when he finished, the woman looked stunning. She went on to buy all the products he recommended. I knew she would never be able to duplicate his results. He probably knew it, too. Unfortunately, she didn't know it and was in for another cosmetic disappointment when she got home. The problem was simple: He had all the professional tools, while she left with inadequate applicators.

Why major cosmetic companies would sell superior cosmetics with inferior applicators had always been an enigma to me. It may have been convenience, or it may have been money. Whatever the reason, women were buying, for example, an eye-shadow compact that would last for two years, but the applicator it was sold with would quickly become inefficient, messy, and might last only two weeks.

Watching that woman in the department store, I decided it was about time women had a chance to apply their makeup like professionals. Every brush, sponge, applicator, and tool that was available to me—the professional—should be available to the consumer, too. While I can't take credit for inventing the lipstick, waterproof mascara, or a better blusher, I can claim to have contributed to making professional brushes and tools available to the consumer.

The reason it was so important to me to put the right brushes and tools in the hands of the consumer is that, in addition to being a makeup artist, I have spent my career *teaching* women how to do their own makeup. As an educator, I recognized that in order for a woman to learn from my lessons, she had to have the same quality brushes and tools that were available to me. If she didn't, nothing I could teach her would enable her to apply her makeup with professional results.

Brushes, applicators, and tools are still fairly new to most women, and they often ask me, "Jerome, do I really *need* all those brushes? Can't I use just a few of them?" My answer is always "Yes, you need every one of them if you want to apply your makeup like a professional." And I'm telling you, too, that you need them. Walk into your kitchen. Open the utensil drawer. Do you really *need* all those knives? If you think you don't, try cutting a steak with a butter knife, or attempt to slice a loaf of hard, crusty bread with a paring knife. The same is true of cosmetic brushes. Each one has its own individual purpose, specially designed for its specific job. You may end up finding that your cosmetic wardrobe includes as many brushes as it does different types of makeup. That's fine. You're on your way to applying cosmetics like a professional.

The Different Types of Makeup Brushes

Fine Eyeliner

The fine eyeliner brush is made of very resilient sable hair. I also refer to this brush as a "needlepoint eyeliner." I use the fine eyeliner brush with pencil eyeliners to smudge color into a fine, indistinct line. I line both the upper and lower lids with a kohl pencil and use the brush to smudge and blend the color.

16

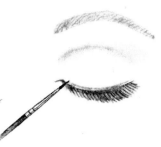

The fine eyeliner brush has many other uses for the professional makeup artist. I still find myself discovering additional uses for this brush. Some of the ways I use the fine eyeliner brush, which you can easily adapt, are as follows.

- Eye shadows today come in an unlimited assortment of colors. Why not take advantage of this infinite scope of color by allowing shadows to do double duty as eyeliners? Many powder shadows, when mixed with a little water, become instant eyeliners. Apply with the fine eyeliner brush. Today's powders have such staying power that they often need not be mixed with water to become eyeliners. Even when dry, applied with the fine eyeliner brush, they function as eyeliners.
- The fine eyeliner brush can be used to create the illusion of diminishing wrinkles and creases when used to apply liquid or cream concealers.
- The fine eyeliner brush is also the ideal finishing tool for perfect lashes. Mascara wands can't get close enough to the roots of the lashes. This is especially obvious on blond eyelashes. The fine eyeliner can be used to paint the base of the lashes with mascara.

Eyeliner Brush

The eyeliner brush is also made from resilient sable hair. It is approximately three times the thickness of the fine eyeliner brush. When wet, the brush comes to a point. This brush performs the same function as the fine eyeliner brush but allows you to draw thicker lines when you want or need them.

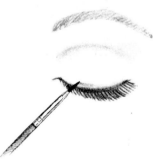

The eyeliner brush is an accessory tool for applying your lip color, because it is thinner than the lip brush. It could be used to achieve fine detail around the mouth. It works especially well in the corners of the mouth.

Eye-Shadow Brush

Made of pony hair for pliability, I call the eye-shadow brush a "doe's foot" because of the way it is shaped. The eye-shadow brush is cut on the bias, tapered down so that its end points can reach the corner of the eye. A good brush should not be too thick—the brushes I use are a maximum of one-eighth inch wide. Although the flat, blunt surface of the brush enables the brush to blend the color, the eye-shadow brush is used primarily to apply eye shadow—particularly on the top eyelid and brow-bone area. You can use the same eye-shadow brush for many shades as long as you can clean the brush between colors—wipe the brush clean on a tissue. Otherwise, you will muddy the colors. It's not necessary, but you might want to invest in two eye-shadow brushes —one for light shadows, another for darker shades.

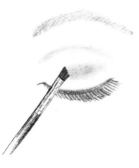

I suggest you use the eye-shadow brushes only when working with powders. I personally don't like to work with creams, but if you do, the sponge applicator is a better tool for the consistency of creams.

Large and Small Shading Brushes

The shading brushes are made out of pony hair, which is soft and pliable but still has a degree of resilience. These brushes fan out at the tip and taper from the flat sides to the center. The main purpose of shading brushes, because they move so well, is blending. They are the brushes that allow you to blend color to the degree of intensity you desire. Both the large and small shading brushes perform the

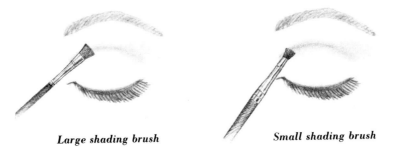

Large shading brush   *Small shading brush*

same function. They are used when contouring, sculpting, and highlighting specific features of the face, such as the nose, jawline, cheeks, chin, and around the eyes. The small shading brush is used for shading small areas, primarily around the eyes, while the large shading brush is meant for shading larger areas of the face. The large shading brush is also used when applying highlighter to the brow bone.

Fluff Brush

The fluff brush is made of goat hair, which is exceptionally soft and pliable. The configuration of the fluff brush is similar to the shading brushes. Its purpose is as a finishing brush, used to dust translucent powder over the eye to set makeup. The fluff brush can be used on any small area of the face that needs dusting with powder. Because of the softness of the goat hair, it glides over the face and doesn't move the shadows or powders.

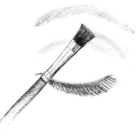

Sponge Applicator

Made of fine, *cosmetic grade* sponge, which is the highest grade of sponge available, applicators are best used for applying liquid or cream eye shadows. Another purpose of the applicator is that it acts almost like an eraser. You can apply a line of color, either eye shadow or pencil, and then almost erase it using the applicator. The shadow that remains creates an illusion of depth and lends drama to the eye.

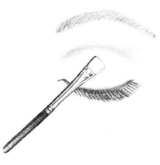

The applicator is also an excellent tool to clean up any minor mistakes in makeup, such as smeared mascara. I use it to clean up any excess eye shadow that may fall on the area below the eye. Whenever I finish doing an eye makeup, I step back, look at my work, and use the applicator to balance the intensity of color—to make both eyes appear even.

I also use applicators for applying concealer under the eyes and for using creams to cover facial imperfections.

Disposable Sponge-Tipped Applicators

These are the same as the sponge applicators, except, as their name implies, you use them a few times and then throw them away. I consider them essential, and I'm sure you will, too. Hygienically, they are superior applicators as they are very sanitary—a crucial factor in preventing eye infections.

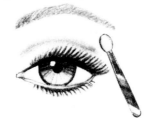

All the things that the regular applicator does, the disposable applicator can do. The difference is, the disposable applicators are inexpensive enough that when they become messy or dirty, you can throw them away. They also come in handy when the applicator that came with your eye-shadow compact must be replaced.

Eyebrow Brushes

The purpose of eyebrow brushes is to brush the brows to their natural shape. You use the eyebrow brush by first reversing the brows and then shaping them back into their natural direction. There are three types of eyebrow brushes:

Boar-Bristle Eyebrow Brush

Made of a stiff, natural fiber, this brush generally has two rows of bristles and resembles a thin toothbrush. Because boar is a natural hair, the bristles are not perfectly even.

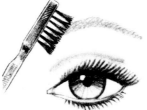

The boar bristle is my personal favorite among eyebrow brushes. In addition to using it to shape the brows, I *automatically* use it to separate lashes after every time I apply mascara. The eyebrow brush removes excess mascara and makes every lash stand out. It can also be used to lighten or darken eyebrows when used to brush on the appropriate light powder or dark eye shadow.

Nylon-Bristle Eyebrow Brush with Comb

This eyebrow brush has nylon bristles and is a brush on one side and a plastic comb on the other. It's used to shape and shade brows and separate lashes just like the boar-bristle brush. In addition, the comb can be used to separate lashes and comb brows into shape.

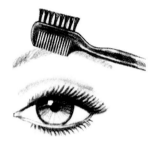

Nylon Tapered Eyebrow Brush

Made of stiff, nylon bristles that taper and are cut on a bias, this brush resembles an eye-shadow brush. I use it to create eyebrows when part of the brow is missing. Using a matching eye shadow (e.g., light brown, dark brown, or a charcoal gray), rub the nylon brush in the eye shadow and, using feathering strokes, you can fashion a natural brow line.

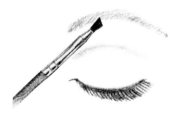

Lip Brush

The lip brush is made of sable hair, which gives it both resilience and control. Approximately one-eighth inch thick, the brush, with lipstick on it, will taper to a blunt tip. Its purpose is to provide smooth, even application of color, with a clean, defined line. The blunt tip is for lining the lips, and the flat—or side—of the brush is used to fill in lip color. Lip gloss, the top coat of lipstick, should also be applied with a lip brush.

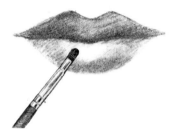

A lip brush allows the professional—and you—to take full advantage of the natural structure and lines of the mouth. It also allows you to make corrections in the shape of the mouth when necessary.

Aesthetically, there is something very elegant about a woman applying lipstick with a lip brush. Practically speaking, it's the only way to get professional-looking results.

Contour Brush

The contour brush is made of goat hair and is more than one-half inch thick. It is a blunt, stubby finishing brush that may also be used for application.

Its chief purpose is shading and highlighting over a large surface such as the cheeks or jawline. Because of the way it is shaped, vigorous movement with the contour brush over a large area creates the illusion of large shadows. The softness and pliability of goat hair aid the brush's blending ability and will not irritate the skin.

The contour brush is used with dark powders, pencils, and creams for contouring, and with light powders, pencils, and creams for highlighting.

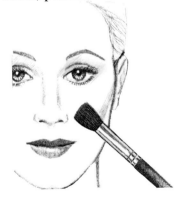

Blusher Brush

A soft, pliable brush made of long (three-quarters to one inch) goat hair, the blusher brush fans out at the top and tapers from the flat sides toward the center. Its sole purpose is to apply and blend blusher. Because of the length of the brush hairs, a stroking motion is made easier. You can create full and even shading along the natural contour of the bone structure. The blusher brush is used on the cheekbone, cheeks, jawline, chin, forehead, and nose.

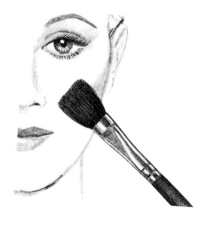

Powder Brush

The powder brush is the largest of all cosmetic brushes. It is made of goat hair approximately one inch thick and over one and a half inches long. The powder brush is a finishing brush used to apply loose or pressed powder to set your makeup. It's used freely over the entire face, neck, shoulders, body, back, and cleavage.

I use as large a brush as possible, and my feeling about powder brushes is the longer, thicker, and fuller, the better.

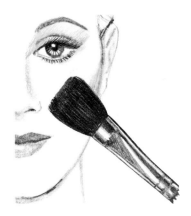

Other Types of Makeup Tools

Sponge Wedges

Triangles of foam, cut in one-inch thickness, these sponge wedges are invaluable to the professional makeup artist. They are used for the blending and application of cosmetics, including foundation.

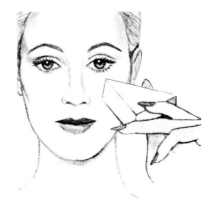

When using sponge wedges for sculpting the face, use the flat side for contouring and the tip for highlighting.

The sponge wedge applies concealer cream or liquid to the under-eye area. The tip of the sponge wedge is ideal for applying foundation to cover small facial imperfections.

The porous sponge will produce a sheer look. I use them to blend powder blushers, and they can also be used as applicators for liquid and cream blushers.

Although sponge wedges can be washed out and reused, they are inexpensive enough so that you may want to start with fresh ones after several makeup applications.

Tweezers

A good pair of tweezers is a sound investment. They are available in three tip varieties—pointed, straight, and slanted; I suggest you choose the pair that you are most comfortable working with.

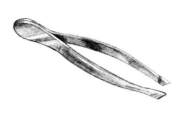

Eyelash Curlers

Many professionals feel an eyelash curler is an essential part of your basic tool kit. I simply do not agree. The truth is, I don't even recommend you own one, unless you have very straight lashes. Most women have naturally curly lashes, and mascara provides additional curl. Use of an eyelash curler can leave you with unnaturally curly lashes. I do not use eyelash curlers when doing a makeup, but if you feel your lashes are just too straight, you can use one with these caveats: (1) Don't curl bottom lashes; (2) don't curl wet lashes—as soon as they dry, they will straighten; and (3) don't curl lashes that already have mascara on them. For each lash you curl, you will probably pull two out!

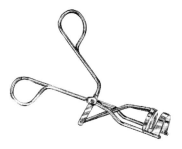

Two-Hole Pencil Sharpener

Some sharpeners are made to accommodate both narrow and wide pencils. This is the kind I suggest you buy. Do not try to sharpen pencils with a knife. When sharpening pencils, always remember to round off the sharp point. This is especially important for eye pencils. *Never go near your eyes with a sharp point of any kind!*

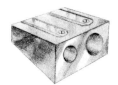

What to Look for
When Purchasing Cosmetic Brushes

Now that you know what kinds of tools you'll need, let's talk about the quality of brushes. There are three parts of the brush that you should examine: the *hair*, the *ferrule*, and the *handle*.

As a professional, I look for the following qualities in a good cosmetic brush.

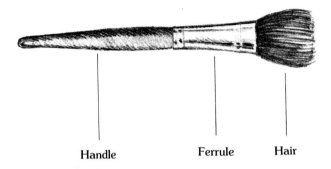

Handle   Ferrule   Hair

Hair

The hair must be natural: pony, goat, sable, or boar bristle. Beware of brushes, except for eyeliner and lip brushes, that claim to be made of 100 percent sable hair. Economically, it's just not feasible. And if it were, it would be inadequate for the job because sable is a very resilient hair. If a powder or blusher brush, which should be made from goat hair, were instead made of sable hair, it would not be soft enough to move and blend the color. The brush hair should be the most appropriate for each brush's function.

Ferrule

This is the metal piece that grips the hair and then connects it to the handle. The best, and most expensive, are made of brass. The strength and hardness of brass hold the hair intact the longest. The less expensive ferrules are aluminum. Because of the softness of aluminum, these ferrules tend to lose their shape after prolonged use and loosen their grip on the hairs.

Handles

Wood-handle brushes are the most desirable and the ones I personally use and recommend. Plastic is less expensive but doesn't offer the grip, balance, or feel of wood. Play with the brushes in your hands to make sure you are comfortable with them.

When purchasing brushes, recognize a basic truth: *Brushes do not last a lifetime.* Like toothbrushes and hairbrushes, they get old, ineffective, and wear out. The set you buy today will eventually have to be replaced. If you notice your brushes losing their hair when new, don't worry—it's a natural process. If they continue to shed, return them—you've been sold an inferior product. If your ferrule becomes detached from the handle, don't panic; instead, do what I do! A little glue will reattach ferrule to handle, making the brush as good as new.

Recognizing that brushes have a limited life-span doesn't mean that they shouldn't receive regular care. This is especially true for sanitary reasons. The majority of all eye infections are from dirty cosmetic tools. Brushes should be tissue-cleaned after each use and deep-cleaned once a week, using the following method.

1. Dip them into rubbing alcohol. They dry quickly, are sterilized, and can't be harmed by the alcohol since they are natural hair.
2. Pat dry with a towel or tissue. Never rub brushes or you will ruin their shape.
3. Stand them upright on their handles, taking care that they do not fall downward onto the hair. Since brushes have a memory of their natural shape, they will return to their original shape after each cleaning.

Now that you know the reason behind each of the tools, I'm sure you'll never again wonder if you really need all of them!

Lay out your brushes and tools in front of you. Face your mirror and get ready for the magic of makeup. As you turn the pages, you'll learn the how-to of the professional. With the right equipment, you'll be able to duplicate the secrets, tips, illusions, and tricks of the trade I've been practicing for over twenty-five years!

2. Contouring and Highlighting

In this book you are going to learn everything you will need to know about applying makeup. You will learn how to choose colors; how to select depth of color; how to use color for maximum effectiveness; how to blend cosmetics until a professional-looking makeup is the result.

This chapter starts the first of your makeup lessons. But before you begin putting cosmetics *on* your face, let's talk about how to properly take your makeup *off* so that you start with a perfectly clean face.

You may have read, or heard a makeup artist insist, that makeup should *always* be removed with cleansing cream. Ideally, this is true; I also recommend removing makeup with cleansing cream. However, the truth is that most women remove makeup with plain soap and water. Each time I give a makeup seminar, I ask how many women wash their faces and take off their makeup with soap and water. Each time, more than 90 percent of the women raise their hands!

Cleansing cream is preferred because it is rich in emollients and it lubricates the skin as it cleanses and removes makeup. Also, the gentle action of a cleansing cream will keep the skin soft and supple. But although in theory you may know you should use a cleansing cream, most women just don't want to change their habits. So instead of insisting that you use only cleansing cream, my advice to you, if you are going to remove makeup with soap and water, is to choose a low pH soap that does not contain detergents or deodorants, which both dull and could irritate the skin. There are many soaps available that, in addition to having a low pH level, contain ingredients that give additional benefits to the skin. For example, translucent soaps contain coconut oil, castor oil, and glycerin, all of which will act to lubricate the skin. If you insist on using soap, always remember to rinse the face well to remove all traces of soap residue.

If you do think you are ready to start a new routine, and would like to switch to a cleansing cream, you may be confused by all the products that are on the market. Finding the one that is right for you is a process of trial and error. There are many inexpensive drugstore brands that have been around for many years that I find quite excellent. There are, of course, also the higher-priced creams that many women like because they are loyal to a particular brand of cosmetics. If you start reading the labels that list the ingredients, you will find that both the expensive and inexpensive creams are basically the same. I personally do not know of any wonder ingredient in a high-priced cleansing cream that would make it so much more expensive. In most cases, you end up paying for more than just the cream; you're supporting the company's image, packaging, and advertising. After trying several different brands, you will be able to determine which cleansing cream is the best for your needs.

The sensitive area around the eye needs special attention when removing makeup. The best way to remove eye makeup is with eye-makeup-remover pads. It is not necessary to buy them; you can create your own. Simply dip cotton pads in mineral oil until they are saturated. Squeeze out the excess moisture and they're ready to use. Both the commercial and homemade pads will remove the eye makeup—especially the difficult-to-remove mascara—and lubricate the eye area. *Never* use a tissue to remove either eye or face makeup. Tissues contain wood fiber and in some cases may irritate the skin.

Once the makeup is removed, be sure to use a skin freshener, which will rid the skin of excess soap or cleansing-cream residue. I do not recommend using a skin freshener with an alcohol content greater than 50 percent. Alcohol plays havoc with the dry areas of the skin, even for women with very oily skin. Instead, choose a freshener with an alcohol content of less than 20 percent. An alternative way to freshen your skin—and my personal favorite—is to soak cotton balls in ice water and freshen your face with these ice-water-soaked cotton balls. Either method will both tighten the skin and give a very refreshing feeling to the face.

Now your face is a clean canvas, ready to respond to the magic of makeup. To prepare your face for the cosmetics that will be applied, you need to apply a protective layer. That protection comes in the form of a moisturizing cream, often referred to as "moisturizer."

The moisturizer you use depends upon which one works best for you. The bulk of all moisturizers are water. In addition, the ingredients listed on a moisturizer will include humectants, emollients, and fragrances. As with cleansing creams, the most expensive is not necessarily the best for you. I would discount or be suspicious of any wonder ingredients.

There are three reasons why it is imperative that you put moisturizer on your face before applying your makeup. The first is the composition and characteristics of facial skin. Facial skin has both oily and dry areas. This *combination skin* means that while your skin may be oily in some areas (usually around the forehead, nose, and chin), it can be dry in other places. Moisturizers put a film on the face and neutralize the overly oily and extremely dry areas of the face, leaving the skin with a balanced surface. Without the balancing provided by a moisturizer, the oily areas of the skin would tend to repel the makeup foundation (the base coat of makeup applied to the face) and the dry spots would act like a sponge and absorb the foundation. The moisturizer acts as a sealer that prevents unwarranted interaction between the facial oils and makeup. It is this sealing action that prevents the foundation from streaking, caking, or turning orange. The foundation rests on top of the film created by the moisturizer.

The second reason for using a moisturizer is to prevent what I call the "peach of today from becoming the prune of tomorrow." As a woman gets older, her skin loses the ability to retain its natural moisture. This is the major reason for wrinkles, lines, and creases. A moisturizer also helps *plump up* the lines and creases of the face, until they seem to disappear. Additionally, it protects the skin from the elements —sun, heat, cold, and pollution.

The third reason for using a moisturizer before you apply makeup foundation is to lubricate the skin. The skin must be lubricated when working with brushes, sponge, fingers, and applicators, in order to make the cosmetics blend on the face. Moisturizer provides that lubrication.

Makeup Foundation

Once your skin has been properly cleansed and moisturized, it is ready to receive a base—or makeup foundation. You apply foundation to even out skin tone and create a smooth canvas for applying cosmetics.

There are three types of foundation that I recommend: *Water-based liquid,* good for oily skin and suitable for evening when you want a *matte* (nonshiny) finish; *oil-based liquid,* good for dry skin and also appropriate for daytime when you want a *dewy,* moist look; and *cream* foundation, good for those who need extra coverage for skin problems like pimples, pockmarks, large pores, burst capillaries, skin discoloration, and age spots.

The color of the foundation you use should be determined by the natural color of your skin. For Caucasian women, there are three basic skin colors: *olive/sallow* complexions; *ruddy/pink* complexions; and *beige* complexions. All makeup foundations have either beige or pink tones. If you have an olive/sallow complexion, you would choose a pink-tinted makeup foundation to take away the sallowness. If your face is naturally ruddy, a beige foundation will tone down the redness. Women who have a naturally beige complexion should take a close look and decide whether the beigeness tends to be ruddy or sallow. Then, choose the appropriate makeup foundation to correct the skin tone.

Black and Hispanic women have many skin-color combinations and there are foundations created specifically for the individual needs of dark skin. I suggest finding a shade that matches your own skin color as closely as possible. In the chapter on ethnic makeup, I will discuss in detail the makeup needs of black and Hispanic women.

Oriental women have sallow skin and therefore should balance the yellowness by choosing a pink-based foundation. Again, in the chapter on ethnic make-up, I will be detailing makeup routines geared to Oriental women.

No matter which ethnic group you belong to, your daytime foundation should match your natural skin tone as closely as possible. For evening, the foundation should always be two shades darker than your natural skin coloring. Most women tend to look better in this darker shade; don't you love the way you look with a tan? Softer evening light allows you to wear a darker foundation without risking the masklike look created when the difference between the foundation and the natural skin tone is so pronounced.

Foundation is applied with your fingers and blended with a sponge wedge. You can either wet the sponge, squeezing out the excess moisture and further drying the sponge on a tissue, or you can start with a dry sponge and let the foundation itself provide the wetness. The wet sponge will help achieve a sheer look.

With your fingertips, place spots of foundation all over the face, being sure to include the forehead, cheeks, chin, nose, and neck. Then, with the sponge wedge, blend up from the neckline into the hairline. *Always* blend in an upward motion, and be sure you cover the entire face—including the lips and eyelids. Blend on the neck and up around the hairline, even putting some foundation

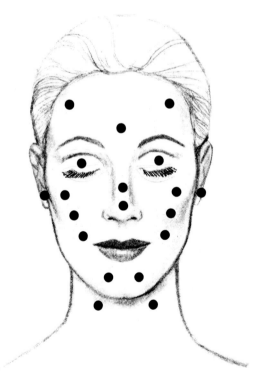

over the entire front of the ears. It is imperative that blending receive a fair amount of your attention to make sure there are no streaks. Many women stop blending along the jawline—which creates an artificial, masklike look. Blending should continue under the chin and on the neck. Blending properly will also prevent the makeup from coming off on your clothes.

Sculpting the Face

Now I'm going to teach you the art of sculpting, highlighting, shading, and corrective techniques that will produce the illusion of the ideal face shape. To me, this is unquestionably the most important aspect of a good makeup—it is the essence of what makeup is all about. Illusion is the heart of makeup. Contouring and highlighting is the key to the creation of illusions. Simply put: *Makeup is magic. Magic is illusion, Therefore, makeup is an illusion.*

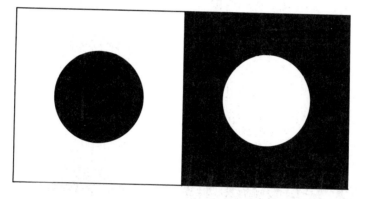

Contouring and highlighting and indeed all aspects of makeup application are based on what is called the "*dark/light illusion.*" It is a very basic art principle: *Dark things look smaller and appear to recede. Light things look larger and appear to come forward.* Look at the sketch of the two circles. If you took a ruler, you would see that the diameters of the circles are identical. Yet when you look at the circles, the black circle appears smaller than the white circle. That is because of the dark/light illusion. Remember this principle. It will influence every decision you make when applying makeup to your face.

Although makeup works on the same dark/light theory as art, it is important to determine what type of art. You are not painting the face; a canvas is flat, but the human face is multidimensional. Makeup is more like sculpture, where the finished product can be viewed from many angles.

You're ready to begin sculpting your face based on a standard ideal. That criteria: The *perfect face* is an oval-shaped face, because it has the most pleasing *width/length ratio.* No matter what your natural face shape is, it is important to discover its width/length ratio.

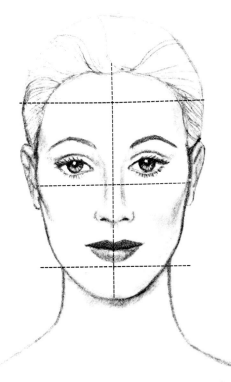

In addition to the criteria of the oval-shaped face, there are standards and ideals for each of the facial features. Within the pages of this book, I will tell you how to create the illusion of ideally shaped facial features. But now, back to the oval-shaped face. Why is it considered the ideal? For centuries it has been deemed the most flattering facial shape. Look at the *Mona Lisa*, other Renaissance paintings, or Egyptian artwork. Most women will have oval-shaped faces.

To measure your face, lift the hair away from your face and look in the mirror. The total length of the face is measured from the tip of the chin to the very center of the forehead at the hairline. The width of the face is measured at three separate places: (1) at the forehead from temple to temple; (2) at the cheekbones from ear to ear; (3) from one end of the jawline to the opposite end. When measuring the face, do not be concerned with actual inches. What is important is determining if your face is longer than it is wide; wider than it is long; or almost equal in length and width. Also important is determining which are the widest and narrowest parts of your face, because that will help you determine your face shape.

Once you know your width/length ratio, you can determine your natural face shape. If it isn't a perfect oval, don't despair! Makeup gives you the ability to create an illusion—and once again *illusion* is the key word. The beauty of cosmetics is that makeup is not a transformation but rather an appearance of change created by illusion. The face that looks back from the mirror will still be yours, but it will be sculpted, highlighted, and enhanced to your maximum advantage.

34

To learn which is your natural facial shape, study the illustrations and read the descriptions of each facial shape. Repeat the process until you are sure you recognize your facial shape. The seven basic facial shapes are:

Round. The face is two-thirds as wide as it is long. The cheeks are the widest part of the face, tapering along the forehead and the jawline.

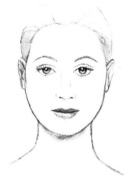

Oblong. The oblong face is longer than it is wide. The cheeks, jaw, and forehead are equal in width.

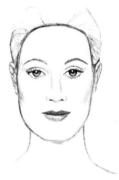

Square. Like the round face, the width is two-thirds or more of the length, but the forehead, jaw, and cheeks are almost equal in width.

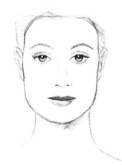

35

Diamond. The widest part of the face is the cheek, and the width is two-thirds or more of the length of the face. Although the dimensions are similar to the round face, the lines of the face—cheek to jaw; cheek to chin—are straight rather than rounded and taper to a narrow forehead and chin.

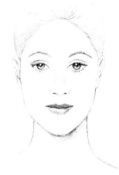

Triangle. The width is generally two-thirds or more of the length of the face. As with the diamond, the lines of the face are straight. The widest part of the triangle-shaped face is at the jaw. The face tapers at the forehead.

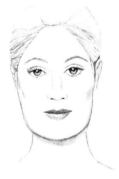

Inverted triangle. The same width/length ratio as the triangle face; the difference is that the widest part of the face is the forehead and the narrowest part is the jaw.

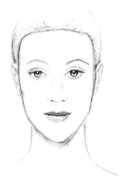

Oval. The width of the oval face is approximately two-thirds of the length. The widest part of the face is the forehead. Curved lines taper gently from the forehead to the chin.

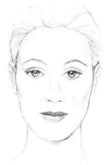

After you have determined your face shape, look into the mirror. Regardless of your facial shape, you will create the illusion of the ideal oval-shaped face by contouring and highlighting. To create an oval shape, simply make an oval with your hands and place it around your face. Keep in mind your face's width/length ratio. If you have a low forehead, start the oval at the hairline. If your forehead is high, begin the oval between the hairline and the eyebrows. If you have a prominent or pointed chin, end the oval at the chinline. However, if your chin recedes, end the oval below the chinline.

Study the oval carefully for a minute. Any part of the face that falls outside the oval, you contour, or shade, with a dark color to make it seem smaller and appear to recede. Any part of the face that falls inside the oval, you highlight with a light color, to bring it forward and give the illusion that it is larger than it actually is.

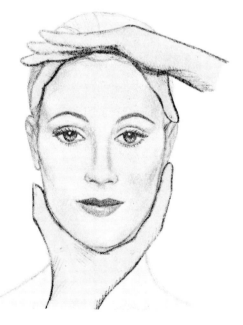

For contouring and highlighting to create the oval-shaped face and to reach the *standards* of all the facial features, you have a myriad of cosmetic products to choose from. Spread your cosmetics in front of you. You will probably find many of the cosmetics you need are already part of your makeup wardrobe.

For contouring, you will need dark cosmetics to make areas of your face appear smaller. You can use:

Dark makeup foundation
Dark blusher (browns, plums, or
    wine)
Dark powdered eye shadow (browns
    and taupes)

Brown pencil
Dark cream shadows

For highlighting areas of the face, light colors will give the illusion of largeness:

Light makeup foundation
Light blusher (pinks, coral, oranges)

White, pink, or white pearl pencil
Any light shade of eye shadow
    (whites, golds, beiges, pinks)

A light cream concealer

Highlight colors can be either matte (nonshiny) or pearlized (iridescent). Pearlized cosmetics act as a double highlighter—both the lightness and the iridescence make areas appear more prominent. This double highlighting effect is very effective in evening makeups.

Now, taking into consideration your natural face shape, follow the step-by-step instructions to contour and highlight your face to create the illusion of an oval-shaped face. In the illustrations, the contoured areas are represented by dark shading. Broken lines indicate areas to be highlighted.

Round face. To minimize the width of the face, use either a dark pencil, dark foundation, etc., to create a shadow on the sides of the forehead. Carry this shadow down the sides of the face and around the jawline. Blend well with a sponge.

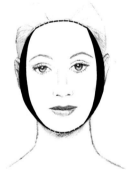

Oblong face. To shorten the length of the oblong face, a dark contour is applied both on the forehead along the hairline and at the tip of the chin. Blend well with a sponge.

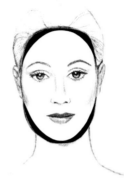

Square face. Shade the corners of the forehead, the cheeks, and the jawline to soften the straight lines of the face. Blend with a sponge or contour brush to give a rounded look to the hairline.

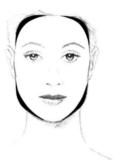

Diamond face. Highlight the sides of the forehead and at the jawline. Blend well with a sponge.

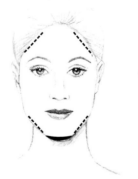

Triangle face. Highlight the temples at the hairline and extend down to the cheekbones to increase the width of the forehead. Contour the lower part of the face under the chin and jawline. Blend well with a sponge.

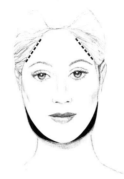

Inverted-triangle face. Darken the areas on both sides of the forehead, down to the top of the ear close to the hairline. Highlight down the sides of the jaw. Blend well with a sponge.

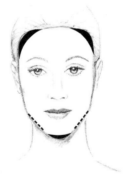

Oval face. Even the oval face needs a little contouring and highlighting if any part of the face falls inside or outside of the oval you make with your hands. Remember, anything outside the oval is contoured. Anything that falls short of the oval is highlighted. (See the diagram on page 65.)

The face that now looks back at you from the mirror should give the illusion of being almost oval-shaped. Now I'll show you how to contour and highlight each feature on your face until you get closer to the standard criteria of the ideal face.

The Forehead

If you have a *low forehead*, you will highlight this area to make the area between the eyebrows and the hairline appear larger. If you have a *high forehead*, you will shade the area to minimize the space between the hairline and the eyebrows.

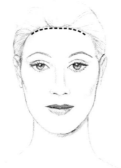

Low forehead, corrected

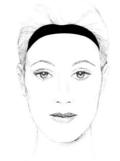

High forehead, corrected

The Chin and Jaw

Now look at your chin. Is it a *prominent or pointed chin?* Then contour the tip of the chin. If the sides of the chin fall inside the oval, highlight the sides of the chin.

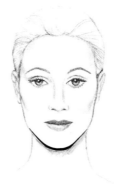

41

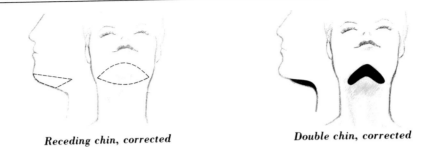

Receding chin, corrected   **Double chin, corrected**

To bring a *receding chin* forward, highlight the tip and sides of the chin. For a *double chin*, apply shadow just under the chin all the way back to the ears, shading under the entire jawbone.

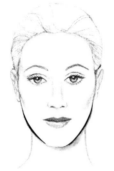

When doing a makeup, I shade practically everyone's jawline—it creates beautiful definition between the chin and the neckline. This step is also included on the technically perfect naturally oval face. When making your oval, shade along the outer part of the jawline and then under the chin on the inner side of the jawline. This look is especially flattering for evening as it provides dramatic definition. The only time you do not shade the inner jawline is in the case of a receding chin. After shading the jawline, blend carefully with a sponge to erase any harsh lines.

The Cheeks

Your goal is to create the illusion of high cheekbones. To achieve your goal, suck in the cheeks and look in the mirror. By sucking in the cheeks, you have created a hollow in the cheeks. Using a contour cosmetic, such as a dark powder or pencil, contour the hollow of the cheekbone, starting in the hollow directly under the center of the eye and working straight back toward the hairline. (See the diagram on page 65.) This will create the illusion of definition to the cheekbones and can be done with any of the face shapes.

Continuing the illusion of high cheekbones, highlight the area directly on the cheekbone. Begin on the cheekbone, directly under the end of the iris closest to the ear and apply color straight back, going right up into the hairline. (See the diagram on page 66.)

The Nose

The nose is probably the least liked feature of the human face. More often than not, women find something to dislike about their noses. There are many different-shaped noses, and most are not the ideal nose. I'll show you how to shade and highlight every imperfection to create the illusion of a more attractive nose.

Broad nose. There are many degrees of a broad nose—from almost flat to slightly broad. For the flat nose, start shading close to the bridge of the nose and shade down the sides. Highlight straight down the center of the nose. For the medium-broad nose, start shading midway between the bridge of the nose and where the nose meets the face. Again, shade down both sides of the nose and highlight down the center of the nose. For the slightly broad nose, begin your shading close to where the nose meets the face. For any broad nose, use a brown pencil to shade the area above the nostrils and at the bottom of the nose.

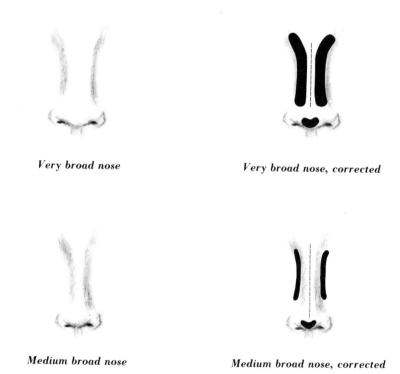

Very broad nose   *Very broad nose, corrected*

Medium broad nose   *Medium broad nose, corrected*

Thin nose. To make the nose appear wider, you can highlight down the sides of the nose. I believe it is best to leave a thin nose alone. When making up a woman with a thin nose, I do not highlight or shade the nose, except to shade the bottom of the nose and the areas above the nostrils.

Nose with a bump. Shade the sides of the nose and shade the bump. Then highlight down the center of the nose, avoiding the bump area.

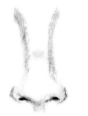

Nose with a bump

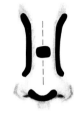

Nose with a bump, corrected

Hook nose. Also known as an aquiline nose; the trick is to diminish the hook by shading the sides and shading the hooked part of the nose.

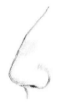

Hook nose

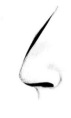
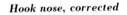

Hook nose, corrected

Short, turned-up nose. Shade the sides of the nose and highlight the center. Highlight all the way down to the tip of the nose. Highlight both the tip of the nose and the area above the nostrils.

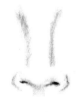

Short, turned-up nose

Short, turned-up nose, corrected

44

Long nose. Shade the sides and, beginning at the middle of the nose, highlight down the center. Shade the entire tip of the nose to make it appear shorter.

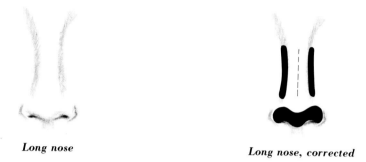

Long nose   **Long nose, corrected**

Bulbous nose. Shade the sides of the nose all the way to the nostrils, and highlight the center of the nose, stopping when you reach the bulbous area. The entire bulbous area should be shaded.

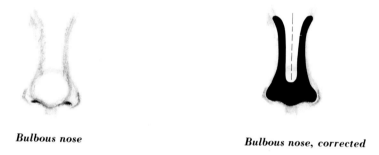

Bulbous nose   **Bulbous nose, corrected**

Crooked nose. Find the area on the tip of the nose that is the prominent bend in the nose. Shade that area. Then, on the top of the nose, highlight the inner curve of the receding area of the nose, which is opposite the prominent bend. Make a straight line down the center of the nose with a highlighter. On the bottom of the nose, shade the prominent area and highlight the receding area.

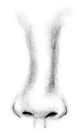 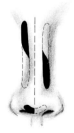

Crooked nose   **Crooked nose, corrected**

The Eyes

I want you to start by taking a good look at your eyes. Look closely into the mirror. Look at the size of your eyes. Examine the space between them. If you can mentally draw a third eye the same size as your own eyes in the space between your eyes, you have *evenly spaced eyes.* If you can draw more than a third eye, then your eyes are *wide-set.* If the space between your eyes is too narrow to draw a third eye, your eyes are *close-set.*

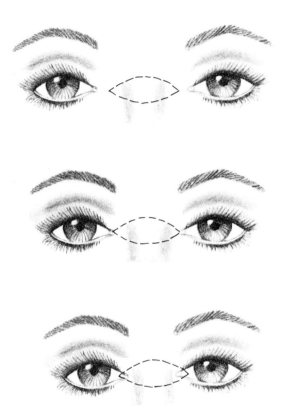

When contouring and highlighting the eyes, please refer to the illustrations of the upper and lower eyelids. Close one eye and feel your upper eyelid. When the eye is closed, it is the area that begins at the nose and ends at the end of the brow bone. Gently run your finger along the eye socket. The half-moon you feel separates the upper eyelid from the brow bone. As you feel the upper lid, you will note that the eye area is concave and convex, rather than flat. For this reason, the dark/light illusion will be used to shape and sculpt your eyes.

46

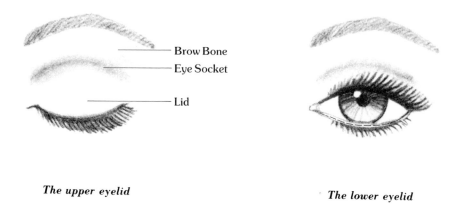

Brow Bone
Eye Socket
Lid

The upper eyelid   *The lower eyelid*

If your eyes are not naturally evenly spaced, you can create the illusion that they are by contouring and highlighting. If you have wide-set eyes, you will shade the first third of the eyelid, closest to the nose. If your eyes are close-set, then the first third of the eyelid will be highlighted. If your eyes are naturally evenly spaced, the decision to either shade or highlight the first one-third of the eyelid becomes a matter of personal choice.

After you have contoured or highlighted your eyes to give them the illusion of being evenly spaced, look in the mirror again to determine if your eyes have any of the following characteristics:

- deep-set
- protruding
- down-slanted
- heavy upper lids
- overly small
- overly large

When you examine your eyes, you may find that they have two characteristics that would technically call for opposite makeup applications. For example, suppose your eyes are both deep-set and widely spaced. To correct the space between your eyes, you would have to use a dark shadow on the inner corner of the upper eyelid. But deep-set eyes require light highlight eye shadows to help bring them forward. The solution is to decide which is the bigger of the two problems and make up your eyes accordingly. Although your eyes may be too widely spaced to be called "ideal," this may not bother you as much as the problem of deep-set eyes.

The next step is to create definition between the upper eyelid and the brow bone, which will bring depth and drama to the eye. As you know by now, this is achieved by contouring the area according to your eye type. The area to be contoured is the *crease* of the eyelid. The crease forms where the upper eyelid and brow bone meet. The crease begins at the inner corner of the eye, close to the nose, and continues until the end of the brow bone. The dark shadow you use to shade this area should be a single line that is smudged. In the illustration of the upper eyelid, the crease is represented by the dotted line. Follow the directions for your eye type.

Close-set eyes. On the upper eyelid, beginning one-third back from the nose, apply a dark line in the crease of the eye, continuing until the end of the brow bone. Smudge the line.

Wide-set eyes. Start the dark line at the innermost corner of the eyelid, close to the nose, and continue it until the end of the brow bone. Smudge the line.

Deep-set eyes. Deep-set eyes have a natural definition, so creating an illusion is unnecessary. This step should be eliminated.

Protruding eyes. Eliminate the shading between the brow bone and the eyelid as it will call attention to the problem of the eyes protruding.

Heavy upper lids. For a woman with heavy upper lids, the eyelid seems to disappear as she opens her eyes. You can create the illusion that when the eye is open there *is* a separation by using a contour between the brow bone and the eyelid. Begin the dark line in the crease of the eyelid on the first third of the eye, closest to the nose, and continue it until the end of the brow bone. This creates an illusion of being able to *see* an eyelid. This step is crucial to any woman with heavy upper lids.

To complete the shaping of your eyes, turn to your eyeliner. Eyeliner is available in cake, liquids, and pencils. I prefer using kohl pencils as they give the softest lines and are the easiest to smudge. Take extra care when using eye pencils and be sure that the pencil you buy is formulated for safe use inside the eye, especially if you have other allergies.

Close-set eyes. The line should start one-third away from the inner corner of the upper eyelid and extend to the end of the eyelid.

Wide-set eyes. The line should be as close as possible to the inner corner of the upper eyelid and should continue until the end of the eyelid.

Deep-set eyes. Eyeliner should be omitted as it will make your eyes appear to recede even further. If you hate to give up your eyeliner, make the line as thin as possible and use a light brown or gray eyeliner instead of a dark brown or black shade.

Protruding eyes. Start the line at the inner corner of the upper eyelid and extend it to the end of the eyelid. Make the line much wider than you usually would when applying eyeliner. Use a medium shade of eyeliner such as a blue or green. Black or brown is too harsh for such a large area. The wider band of color, in a medium shade, looks like a combination of eyeliner and eye shadow. Its effect is to shade the area without giving it an overly harsh look.

Down-slanting eyes. Eyeliner is the perfect cosmetic to correct down-slanting eyes. To create an illusion of reshaping the eye, start at the inner corner of the upper eyelid for wide-set eyes, and one-third away from the inner corner for close-set eyes. Rather than drawing a straight line, make the line on an upward incline toward the end of the eyelid. Using a sponge-tipped applicator, smudge the line in an upward movement toward the brow. Smudge until the line is almost erased and only a shadow remains. On the lower eyelid, apply liner and again proceed to smudge with a sponge-tipped applicator upward toward the brow. This gives the illusion of an upward turn to the eyes.

Small eyes. Line the upper eyelid as you normally would, depending upon the spacing of your eyes. If you have small eyes, never put dark liner on the platform of the lower lid as it will make the eyes appear even smaller. Instead, use a blue pencil on the platform of the lower lid—represented by the dotted area in the illustration of the lower eyelid. This blue pencil will open up the eyes.

Large eyes. Apply eyeliner to the upper eyelid, taking into account the spacing of your eyes. Large eyes can have dark liner put on the platform of the lower lid and it will work to an advantage. It will still make the eyes appear smaller, but large eyes can make the sacrifice in size in exchange for the depth and drama the eyes will acquire.

For all eyes. No matter what type of eyes you have, never frame your eyes with eyeliner. This will give the eye a closed look and make them appear smaller. There should be a slight separation between the end of the liner on the upper lid and the liner on the lower lid. The outside corners of both lids should not be ringed with eyeliner.

The Lips

A perfectly colored mouth gives the face a balanced look. Lip color can also be used to correct any minor imperfections in lip size, shape, and color pigment. Each lip shape has its own rules for makeup application. Before applying lip color, make sure your lips have received a base coat of foundation. It will make the lip color last longer and will also even out any discolorations in your lips, making sure that you get the *true* shade of your lip color.

Study your lips in the mirror and decide which type of lips you have, based on the sketches and descriptions below. In chapter 6, I will be giving extensive instructions for perfectly made-up lips. Here, I want you to concentrate on corrective makeup techniques for your lips.

Even lips. The top and lower lip are evenly proportioned. If even, you can choose any shade of lipstick, dark or light, and also have the option of either using pearlized or regular formulas of lipstick.

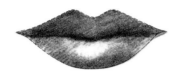

Thin lips. To make thin lips appear fuller, line the entire outer ridge of the upper and lower lips with a white pearl or light pencil. Don't start beyond the outer ridge of the lips. You cannot draw on fuller lips; they will look artificial and clownlike. Fill in the lips with a pearlescent shade of lip color. The effect of the lightness and iridescence will be to make the lips appear fuller.

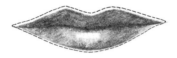

Small mouth. Make an "O" with your mouth. On the outer ridge of the "O," at each corner of the mouth, place a tiny dot of your lipstick color. By placing small dots on the outer ridge, you will create the illusion that the mouth extends further than it actually does. Fill in lips with lip color.

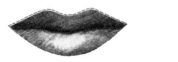 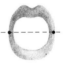

Large mouth. Stop your lip color just a fraction of an inch before the ends of the mouth. Use a darker lipliner to minimize the fullness of the mouth, and fill in lip color in a corresponding shade.

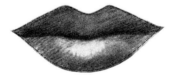

Mismatched lips. This can either be a combination of a fuller upper lip and a thin lower lip or a thin upper lip and a fuller lower lip. Apply lipstick to each as befits that particular lip shape. That means using light shades, starting on the outer ridge for the thin lips and a darker corresponding shade, starting on the inner ridge for the fuller lip.

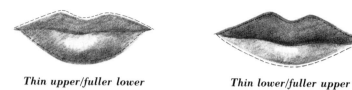

Thin upper/fuller lower   *Thin lower/fuller upper*

Down-turned mouth. Look in the mirror and make an "O" with your mouth. Place tiny dots of your lipstick color in each corner of your mouth. Shade lips in with lip color. The dots on the corners will *lift* the downward motion of the mouth. This trick actually works on all mouth shapes and gives the lips a pleasing, upturned look.

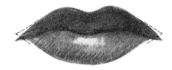

Bow lips. Bow lips are the one exception where you can draw on a fuller mouth, because the natural lipline is already there on the center of the mouth. The lipline recedes rapidly from the center, creating an unusual arch. From the center of the mouth, draw a straight line to the corners of the mouth and fill in the bowed area with lip color.

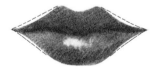

Crooked lips. You must be very careful when trying to compensate for a crooked mouth. The trick is to correct as much as possible without overcorrecting, which ends up looking artificial. In most cases, I suggest you follow the mouth's natural lipline.

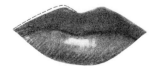

3. Blusher

With the application of blusher, you begin to put cosmetics on your face that, in addition to sculpting the face, will leave noticeable color. Before applying color to the face, remember:

Everything you put on the face has to have a very definite reason for being there. Nothing is ever applied indiscriminately. What you choose to put on your face, the color you select, the depth of color and where it is applied must have a definite reason for being there.

Blusher is possibly the most misunderstood and misused cosmetic. The principle of blusher is based entirely on the dark/light illusion theory. You will need at least two blushers, never just one shade, to do the job correctly. You will need a dark blusher for contouring and a light blusher for highlighting.

Blushers are available in powders, creams, and gels. As I've said before, I work only with powders; this is especially true when I'm working with blushers. Powders are able to give a soft, natural texture. Cream blushers generally do not blend as well, are not as easy to apply, and, most important, do not afford you the control that powders do. Additionally, creams do not look as good on women with problem skin and large pores. Powder will glide over these problems while creams seem to call more attention to them by clogging the large pores.

How to Apply Blusher

In working with all powders, you should get into the habit of using your hand or a tissue as a palette. This is what I, as a professional makeup artist, do. I prefer using my hand as a palette because the color that comes directly from the brush to the face is much too intense. Powders are very concentrated, very intense, and by brushing the color back and forth on the hand, you can adjust the shade until you've reached the intensity you want for your face.

Begin by using a dark blusher for a contour. Go over the areas you contoured when shaping your face, everything that falls outside the oval, shading lightly with the dark blusher. Next, suck in the cheekbones. Envision an imagi-

53

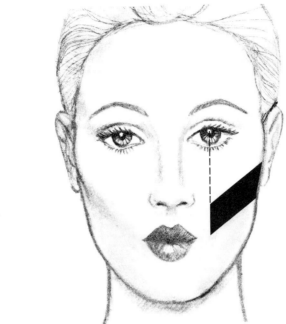

*How to apply
dark blusher*

nary line that starts downward directly under the center of the eye. Extend this line to the hollow of the cheek, below the cheekbone. Begin applying your dark blusher from this spot in an upward motion into the hairline. Blend well with a sponge.

Next, turn to your light blusher, whose purpose is to highlight. The easiest way to remember where to highlight with blusher is to remember that blusher should look like the natural kiss of the sun. When you're out in the sun, the areas that respond to the sun first are the tip of the nose, cheeks, forehead, and chin. This is just where you should apply your light blusher with the blusher brush. Remember to blend well with a sponge every time you apply color to the face.

- Smile—apply the light blusher directly on the full part of the cheekbones, starting directly under the center of the eye and moving upward and into the hairline.
- Place some light blusher right on the tip of the chin. If you have a protruding chin, then you should use a dark blusher.
- Apply light blusher to the tip of the nose. If you have a long nose, use a dark blusher instead.
- A light blusher should be used in the center of the forehead between the eyebrows and the hairline.

The rule for *dark* blusher application always remains the same, but there are two specific cases where the rules for *light* blusher application change. The first case is the woman with a round face. Because the width/length ratio of the round face is almost equal (the area from chin to forehead and from cheek to cheek are almost the same), the illusion of greater length is needed. Use the light blusher to achieve this illusion. While looking straight ahead, envision an imaginary line extending downward from the outer end of the iris to the cheekbone. Apply light blusher directly on the cheekbone to create a line past the eye going directly up to the top of the temple.

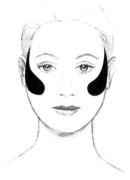

The second case where you change the blusher application is for an oblong face. The forehead-to-chin length is so much greater than the width from cheek to cheek that some width is needed. To achieve the illusion of width, smile —looking straight ahead from the end of the iris and starting on the cheekbone, work straight back toward the center of the ear.

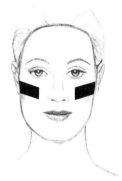

After the application of blusher, it is imperative to blend well with the sponge until a soft, nondefinite line results. You should never be able to tell where the blusher begins and where it ends.

Blushers are available in two formulas: matte, which is a flat, sheer, nonshiny color; and iridescent—gleaming and glittery. Iridescent blushers are primarily used for evening and they should be used only as highlight blushers. Mattes, depending on whether they are dark or light, can work both as contour or highlight blushers.

Although your color range in blushers is unlimited, you should have a color plan or monochromatic scheme in mind when applying makeup. Blusher should complement the color on your eyes, lips, etc.

A final word about blushers. Often, women seem to be applying blusher several times during the day or evening. This is because it was not applied properly the first time. The only cosmetic you should need to reapply is lipstick—because you are constantly eating it off. Blusher, applied the way I outline above, should last with one application until you remove your makeup.

4. Eyes

I'm going to show you, step by step, how to make up your eyes to their maximum advantage. Once again we'll be working on the dark/light–illusion principle, but first I'd like to say something about the term *eye shadow*. Although it is universally accepted that every shade from white to off-black is an eye shadow, and I myself refer to all shades as "eye shadows," in truth "eye shadow" is a misnomer. Working with the dark/light principle, all *light*-colored eye shadows are in reality eye *highlighters*. And dark shades are truly *eye shadows*.

Remember how, when you applied foundation to your face, I told you to make sure to cover the entire eye area as well? The foundation you applied will act as a base to receive the many different shades you will apply to the eye area. It will also provide an even skin tone, assuring you of getting the true tones of the eye shadows and eyeliners.

Take a step back and look at your eyes in the mirror. Examine the structure of your eyes. Are they wide-set, close-set, evenly set, deep-set, down-slanting, or protruding? If you need to, refer back to the eye sketches in chapter 2, "Contouring and Highlighting." Depending upon which type of eyes you have, you will apply eye shadow accordingly.

To begin making up your eyes, I want you to look at your eyelid and mentally divide it into three parts, beginning at the nose and finishing at the end of the eye socket. My theory is to apply eye shadow *vertically*, rather than horizontally, in view of the fact that the eye is multidimensional. Vertical application of eye shadow allows you to play up the convex and concave areas of the eye. Feel for the brow bone from the beginning of the nose to the end of the eye socket. You will begin working from the brow bone down to the eyelashes. Now once again envisioning the eyelid in three parts, begin the first third of the eyelid.

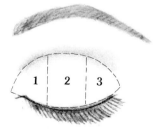

Close-set eyes. Choose a light-colored eye shadow for the first one-third of the eyelid, closest to the nose, to create an illusion of eyes being further apart.

Wide-set eyes. For the first third of the eyelid, select a dark eye shadow to make eyes appear closer together.

Evenly spaced eyes. You have the option of using a dark or light shadow on the first third of the eyelid.

Protruding eyes. These eyes have unique makeup application and will be dealt with separately in this chapter.

Deep-set eyes. Please refer to the section on deep-set eyes later in this chapter.

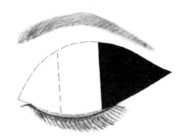

For all eyes, the center of the eyelid gets a very light highlight eye-shadow shade.

On the last third of the eyelid, we choose a darker eye-shadow shade. Feel along the last third of the eyelid toward the end of the brow bone. Using an eye-shadow brush, follow that line until the end of the socket. Then, going back to right above the lashes, make a "V." Fill in the V area with the dark color.

With the large shading brush, evenly blend the three colors together to achieve the effect of one, undefined color. You should not be able to tell where one shade ends and the next shade begins.

Over and over I am going to tell you that your choice of color is unlimited; but when choosing from the wide range of shadows, select colors that complement one another. Conflicting shades (pinks and greens, browns and blues) make it more difficult to achieve a monochromatic, one-color look than if you choose, for example, brown, gold, and plum eye shadows. Think about most eye-makeup compacts you have purchased. You'll notice they are sold in color *families*.

The next step, now that color has been applied to the eyelid, is to create a definition between the brow bone and the eyelid. This creates depth and lends drama to the eye.

Using an eye-shadow or small shading brush, apply a dark, thin line of shadow in the *crease* of the eyelid—not on the brow bone and not on the eyelid. The line is applied in the following manner:

Even and wide-set eyes. Begin the line in the crease of the eye above the first third of the eyelid and continue it until the end of the eyelid.

58

Close-set eyes. Begin the line in the crease, starting at the center of the eyelid and continuing until the end of the eyelid.

This step can be accomplished with any dark color (brown, plum, taupe, gray, dark blue, dark green) and either a powder eye shadow or eye pencil will do the job. After application, use a large shading brush and blend up toward the outer end of the eye.

As I mentioned in chapter 2, "Contouring and Highlighting," one of the most common problems when applying eye makeup is when the eyes have what is called a "heavy upper lid." Normally, when the eye is open, it is still possible to see a portion of the upper lid. However, if you have heavy upper lids, the eyelid seems to disappear completely into the brow bone. There are varying degrees of heavy upper lids. I have noticed that as women mature they may develop this problem as the skin on the eyelids loses its elasticity and becomes crepey.

The cosmetic correction for heavy upper lids is to apply makeup for your eye type as explained earlier, except when creating the definition between the lid and the brow bone. If you have heavy upper lids, the line in the crease of the eye should be accentuated. It should be a thicker line, drawn in the crease of the eye and thick enough to touch slightly on the brow bone and slightly on the eyelid.

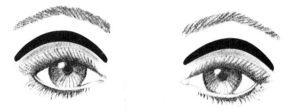

The last eye shadow to be applied is a highlighter on the outer portion of the brow bone. The shadow should be a very light highlighter such as a white, light pink, or light gold, and should be used very sparingly. The only time you change this step is if you have a protruding brow bone. Then the brow bone should get a *contour* shade.

Eyeliner

The purpose of eyeliner is to bring depth to the eyes, make eye lashes appear longer and darker, and reshape the eye. That's quite a job for a very thin line that's barely noticeable! But it illustrates that makeup, applied properly, need never be excessive to be effective. Eyeliners are available in liquids, cakes, and pencils. I prefer a kohl pencil. It is a charcoal pencil, similar to an artist's pencil, and will smudge easily. As always when working with eye pencils, make sure the point is not too sharp by smoothing it with your finger.

Upper Eyelid

Close-set eyes. Start the line at the beginning of the center of the eyelid and bring it to the outer end of the eyelid, staying close to the base of the lashes.

Even and wide-set eyes. Start the line at the beginning of the first third of the eyelid and continue it until the end of the eyelid.

My theory about eyeliner is that by creating a thin line with a kohl pencil and smudging that line with an eyeliner brush or sponge-tipped applicator, you can still achieve all the effects of eyeliner without having a thick, dark, exaggerated line that looks both harsh and hard. You can use gray, brown, black, or any dark color (e.g., navy blue, plum) as an eyeliner.

To reshape the eyes and give them a slightly upturned look, apply the liner from the beginning to end of the eyelid, but rather than following the natural line, make the line peak upward on the latter part of the last third of the eyelid. Now, place your finger at the end of the brow bone. You should be able to feel an indentation. When blending the eyeliner with a brush or sponge-tipped applicator, blend upward at the end of the brow bone into that definition, toward the eyebrow. Then, almost erase the line with a sponge-tipped applicator, leaving only a slight shadow. This will create an illusion of the eyes having an upturned look.

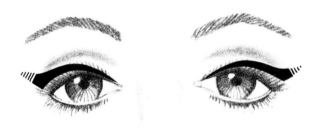

Lower Lid

Eyeliner on the lower eyelid is used for the same reason as on the upper lid—that is, it's applied to bring depth and drama to the eye and to reshape the eye. In addition to the area directly under the lower lashes, eyeliner can be applied to the platform of the lower lid.

Dark eyeliner (black, gray, brown, navy), when applied to the platform of the lower lid, makes your eyes appear smaller. I recommend that only women with large eyes apply an eyeliner to this area. Large eyes can trade off the apparent decrease in size for the depth and drama the dark liner will provide.

To make any size eyes appear larger, but small eyes in particular, line the platform of the lower lid with a light blue pencil. The blue acts like a mirror for the whites of the eyes. This illusion makes the whites of the eyes appear both whiter and larger, which in turn makes the entire eye appear larger. The beauty of this makeup trick is that it works on all eyes shapes, eye colors, skin colors, and age groups.

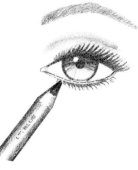

To line the lower lid, use a kohl pencil, liquid, cake eyeliner, or powdered eye shadow below the platform of the lower lid, lining the entire lower lid area no matter if your eyes are evenly, closely, or widely spaced.

Using an eyeliner brush or sponge-tipped applicator, smudge the color back and forth, softening the line. Moving upward while smudging, again smudge into the indentation at the end of the brow bone. Do not frame the upper and lower eyelids with eyeliner as this will make eyes appear smaller. There should be a slight separation between the upper and lower lines.

Protruding Eyes

For the steps that I have described, protruding eyes seem always to be the exception. Protruding eyes are actually quite uncommon, and when they do occur, it may be due to an overactive thyroid. However, if you have slightly protruding eyes, this makeup will help create the illusion that your eyes do not protrude.

Protruding eyes are made up by a line of dark eye shadow approximately one-quarter inch thick drawn at the base of the upper lashes. The line is a straight one drawn from the beginning to the end of the eyelid. Do not highlight the brow bone and do not create a definition in the crease of the lid. Apply the light blue pencil on the platform of the lower lid, and eyeliner on the lower lid, below the platform.

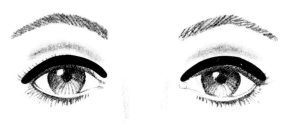

Deep-set Eyes

Deep-set eyes should always get light-highlight eye shadows to make the eyes appear to come forward. Use a light eye shadow for the first third of the eyelid and a very light-highlight shadow for the center of the eyelid. On the last third of the eyelid, place a medium-light shade and make the "V," filling it with the medium-light shade of color.

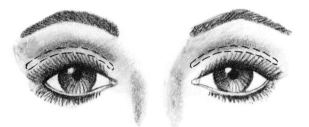

If you have deep-set eyes, *do not* add a dark shadow in the crease of the eye between the brow bone and the eyelid for added definition. Deep-set eyes have this definition naturally. I personally do not recommend lining the upper lid with a dark eyeliner, as eyeliner gives added depth to the eye. You can, however, apply a blue pencil to the platform of the lower lid to make the eyes appear larger.

Mascara

Lashes are the frame of the eye. The purpose of mascara is to make eyelashes thicker, darker, and longer. Think of each of your eyes as a beautiful painting that should be surrounded by an equally beautiful frame. The proper result of mascara is that each lash should be coated, yet remain separate and individual.

The key to applying mascara properly is to make every lash count. Mascara is available in both waterproof and nonwaterproof formulas. I recommend that you not use the waterproof mascaras. The difference between the two types is that waterproof mascara has more paraffin in it. Paraffin is a wax, and it causes the lashes to clump together. Unless you plan to become the next Esther Williams, nonwaterproof mascara will be more than adequate.

I also recommend that you stay away from black mascara. It can look very hard and harsh. Instead, choose an off-black, brown/black, or brown shade of mascara. Colored mascara (greens, blues, etc.) are very artificial-looking and I never recommend them.

Mascara is available in cake form, which you wet and apply with a special brush, or in a cream form contained in a cylinder, accompanied by a wand. The automatic cylinder with the wand is the most widely used type of mascara and the form I recommend. The trick to using this type is first to remove the excess mascara that forms a glob on the tip of the wand. It is this excess that causes mascara to smear on the brow bone, under the lashes, etc. Before beginning to apply mascara, simply wipe the excess on a tissue.

Applying Mascara to the Upper and Lower Lashes

Most women hold the wand flat and work in an up-and-down motion. I suggest that, instead, you hold the wand upright and move from side to side. Take the pinky finger of the hand that holds the wand and rest it on your cheek to steady your hand and provide added control. This method allows you to coat each lash separately, coat both the tops and undersides of the lashes, and get to the roots of the lashes. This is especially important for blondes and redheads with fair-colored lashes.

After applying a coat of mascara, but before it dries, take an eyebrow brush or an eyebrow comb and separate the lashes, removing any excess mascara. Too many coats of mascara result in caked lashes. Two coats are usually all that is needed. In between coats of mascara, powder lashes with translucent powder. This will help the mascara to cling to the lashes. On the lower lashes, work from the inner corner to the outer corner of the eye. Again, separate lashes and remove excess mascara with an eyebrow brush or comb.

In most cases, proper application of mascara will provide thick, attractive lashes that are naturally curled. As I said earlier, I generally do not recommend

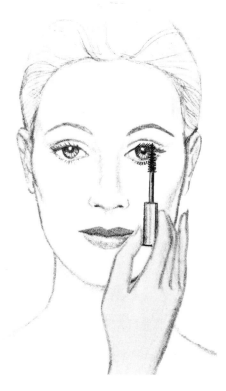

using an eyelash curler except for those women who have very straight lashes. If you feel your lashes need curling, refer to chapter 1 for instructions on the proper use of an eyelash curler.

An alternative to mascara is eyelash dying. A dye is applied to the lashes to keep them dark. Many women choose to have their eyelashes dyed in the summer when water sports make nonwaterproof mascara impractical. Also, blondes and redheads, born with very fair lashes, find eyelash dying a way to have noticeable lashes without applying mascara. If you decide to have your eyelashes dyed, it *must* be done by a reputable, licensed cosmetologist in a professional beauty salon. I also recommend that, prior to having your eyelashes dyed, you take a *sensitivity test*, in which the cosmetologist will apply the dye to a patch of skin on the arm.

The Steps to a Perfect Makeup

Where to apply contour and/or highlight

1 or 2

1 or 2

2

3

2

1

2

1 or 2

2

1 or 2

Key

1 Contour
2 Highlight
3 Under-eye concealer

Note: Where the key shows a choice of a contour (1) or highlight (2) cosmetic, choose the cosmetic that will give your features the illusion of being ideally shaped.

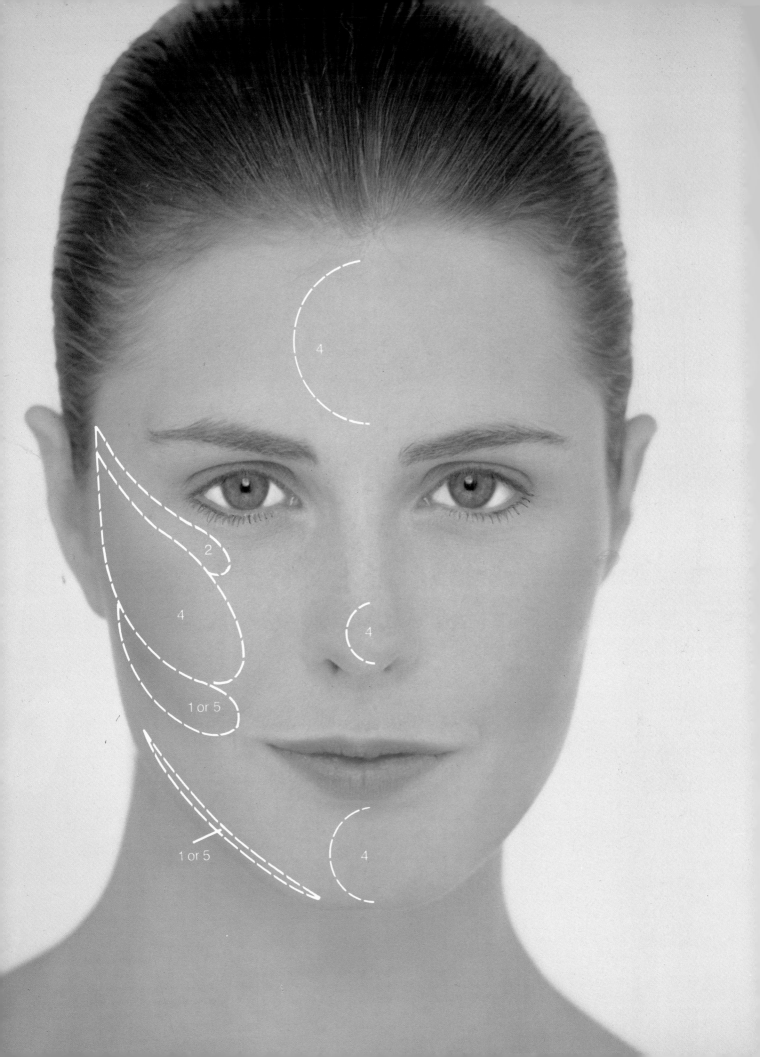

◀ *Where to apply blusher*

▼ *Where to apply makeup*
   for your eyes

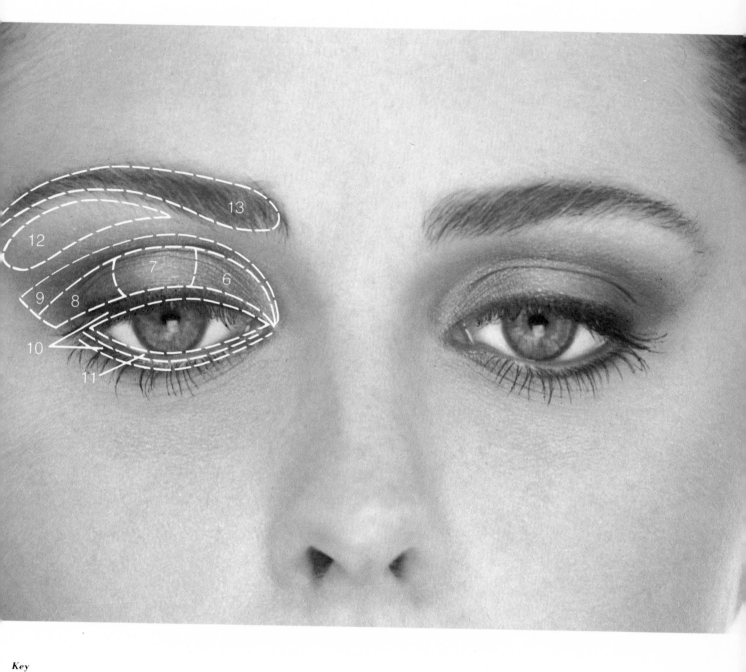

Key

1 *Contour*
2 *Highlight*
3 *Under-eye concealer*
4 *Light blusher*
5 *Dark, contour blusher*
6 *Light eye shadow for
   close-set eyes, dark eye
   shadow for wide-set eyes,
   dark or light eye shadow
   for evenly spaced eyes*
7 *Highlight eye shadow on
   the center of the upper
   eyelid*
8 *Dark eye shadow for the
   outer third of the upper
   eyelid*
9 *Eye contour in the crease
   of the eye socket*

10 *Eyeliner on the upper and
    lower eyelids*
11 *Lining the platform of the
    lower eyelid with a light
    blue pencil*
12 *Highlight on the brow
    bone*
13 *Properly shaped eyebrows*

*Note: Where the key
shows a choice of a
contour (1) or highlight
(2) cosmetic, choose the
cosmetic that will give
your features the illusion
of being ideally shaped.*

Where to apply makeup
for your lips

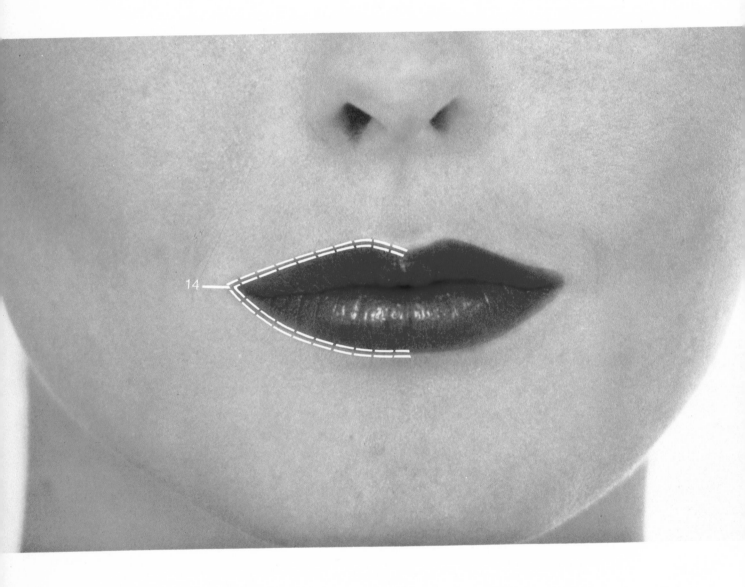

5. Eyebrows

The eyebrows form but a small part of the face, and yet
they can darken the whole of life by the scorn they express.

—Demetrius

If I had to pick one single feature that gives a definite expression, it would be the eyebrows. They can give your face a sad, happy, quizzical, angry, stern, or surprised look. So how you tweeze and shape your brows is critical if you don't want to give the world the wrong impression!

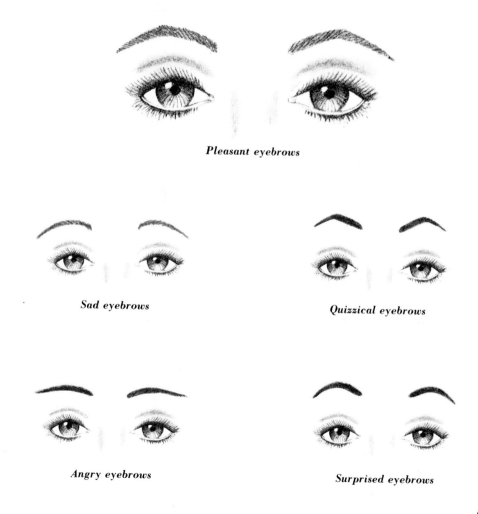

Pleasant eyebrows

Sad eyebrows

Quizzical eyebrows

Angry eyebrows

Surprised eyebrows

Let's begin by examining the proper shape for the eyebrow. The ideal brow shape for your face relates directly to the spacing between your eyes and nose. To determine this shape, first brush your brows in reverse to elongate the hairs, then smooth them in their natural direction. The balanced brow is fullest at the inner portion (A); the outer half (B) tapers to a slender line (C).

Looking at the illustration, and at your own eyebrows in the mirror, note that the brow begins at point A directly over the inner corner of the eye. The arch of the brow is at point B directly over the outer edge of the iris of the eye. The brow ends at point C where a line slanted from the side of the nose past the outer corner of the eye meets the brow. From points A to C should be a straight line. Both ends of the brow touch line D. Point B should be one-quarter inch above line D. Neither end is higher or lower than the other.

This is the ideal shape you are after, and tweezing the eyebrows is the best method to obtain it. Although from decade to decade different types of eyebrows are in vogue—be they pencil-thin or lushly thick—the essential shape remains the same.

As I discussed earlier, there are three types of tweezers: straight, slanted, and pointed. Choose the one you are most comfortable working with.

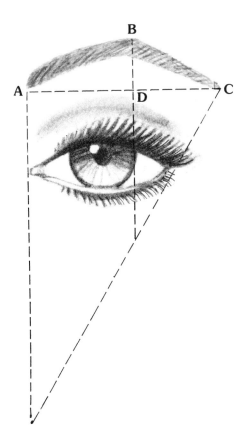

How to Tweeze

- Always wash the eye and eyebrow area first and dip the tweezers in alcohol to remove any dirt. Again and again I am going to stress the importance of keeping tools and cosmetics as clean as possible. It's your best bet against infection.
- Never tweeze eyes immediately before going out as a certain amount of irritation and puffiness may occur. You're better off tweezing the night before, when a good night's rest will give your skin a chance to recover from any swelling or soreness.
- An excellent way to anesthetize the area you are tweezing is to freeze it with an ice cube.
- Never tweeze eyebrows from the top. Always work from the bottom, tweezing one line at a time, until your reach the desired shape.

Let me add that if you are uncomfortable tweezing your own brows, you have the option of having them professionally done. And I stress the word *professionally*. Go to a reputable beauty salon and have your eyebrows shaped by a licensed cosmetologist.

In addition to tweezing there are other ways to keep your eyebrows looking their best. To shape and train brows, use an eyebrow brush and reverse the brows first, then shape them in their natural direction. For added hold, add a light misting of hair spray to the eyebrow brush. If you keep repeating the process, eyebrows, like hair, will be trained to stay in the direction you want them. An alternative to hair spray is clear lip gloss.

Your eyebrows, like every other feature on your face, should appear balanced. They should not be too dark or too light in relation to your hair coloring and complexion. If your brows are too dark, brush some light eye shadow on the eyebrow brush when shaping them into place. If they are too light, use the same process with dark shadow. Sometimes, whether from poor tweezing, habits, accidents, etc., all or part of the eyebrow is missing forever. You can create eyebrows with cosmetics, although I don't recommend drawing brows on with an eyebrow pencil. The shiny, greasy composition of the pencils creates eyebrows that are harsh and unnatural; to me, that is a totally artificial look. But there is a way to create natural-looking brows:

1. Use a nylon-tipped eyebrow brush. While the nylon-tipped eyebrow brush is best suited to creating natural-looking brows, you can also use an eye-shadow brush for this purpose.
2. Choose an eye shadow that blends with the natural color of the hair.
3. Instead of drawing on brows, work on top of the natural brow and, with soft, feathery strokes, improve the shape of the natural brow. I've found that the taupes are the best shades of eye shadow for creating eyebrows. They seem to work on almost all brow colors and have a very neutral quality to them.

71

4. Work very lightly, using the hand as a palette for control, and build the color slowly.
5. To finish, go back to the eyebrow brush to make sure the eye shadow is carefully blended with your brow.

Using this method, you create the illusion that the brows are natural hair rather than drawn on.

Properly shaped, well-cared-for eyebrows are a matter of simple good grooming. Even if you do not wear makeup, your eyebrows should always be attractively shaped. In the overall picture of your makeup routine, perfectly shaped eyebrows will help achieve the goal you're after—a professional-looking makeup.

6. Lips

Fact: The single largest-selling item in the multibillion-dollar cosmetic industry is lipstick. Lipstick seems to hold a fascination for women unequaled by any other cosmetic. Lipstick is usually the first item a little girl takes from her mother's cosmetic bag to experiment with. As adults, lipstick is usually the one makeup item that women will not leave the house without wearing.

It's been my experience that the majority of women have very attractive mouths. The mouth is also the easiest facial feature to correct with makeup, because the natural guidelines—the liplines—are already there to follow. Achieving an attractively made-up mouth is one of the simplest makeup applications to learn.

Just like the other features on the face, the lips need to be *prepared* to receive lip color. Start by applying a moisturizer to the lips, followed by a base of foundation. This base coat of foundation will even out your own natural lip color to assure you of getting the true shade of the lipstick.

The complaint I hear most often about lipstick is "The lipstick I buy never looks the same on my lips as it did in the store." This is because most women test lipstick on the backs of their hands, not on their lips. The only way to achieve the true shade of the lipstick on your lips is to prevent your natural lip color from coming through and distorting the shade of the lipstick. A base coat of foundation solves this problem.

A base of foundation will also help lipstick to stay on the lips longer. Although lipstick does need to be reapplied during the day, as it is constantly being eaten off, foundation helps the color *cling* to the lips.

One of the biggest mistakes women make when applying lipstick is to apply the color directly from the lipstick instead of using a lipliner or a lip brush. Applying the color straight from the stick will result in an uneven, nondefinitive line. It is only with a lipliner pencil or lip brush—preferably a sable lip brush—that you can achieve the control necessary for perfectly made-up lips.

When choosing a lipstick color, you should have a preconceived idea of the color scheme of your makeup. You should try to work within a color-coordinated family: For example, if your blusher is pink, your lipstick should also be in the pink family. Clothes have a bearing on the shade you choose, as do hair color, skin color, and mood. While a vivid fuchsia mouth might seem a bit much for the office, it might be just the color for a night out!

How to Apply Lip Color

Above, I suggest using a sable lip brush because the hair is resilient enough to make the definitive lines you're looking for. Make sure your brush has been tapered properly. When lipstick is applied to the brush, the hairs should form a blunt tip. You use the blunt tip of the brush to outline the lips, using very little lip color on the brush. Be especially careful to use lip color sparingly when working with dark colors.

To make sure the lipstick stays within the boundaries of the lipline and doesn't bleed into the corners and creases of the mouth, first line the lips with a lipliner. The purpose of lipliner is to give a more definite line to the lips. Lipliner is just lipstick with a very heavy paraffin (wax) content. Wax makes the lipstick less likely to run. This is especially useful for more mature women, whose lipstick tends to bleed into the creases and corners around the mouth.

Here is a surefire way for beginners to make up their lips perfectly. Look at your face in the mirror. Looking closely at your nose and lips, look at the lines that begin directly underneath the nostrils and continue to the outer ridge of the lips. Where the lines meet the ridge of your lips, make a small dot with your lip color. On the lower lip, place two tiny dots of lip color, directly under those that appear on the upper lip. Next, make an "O" with your mouth and place a tiny dot of lip color in each corner of the mouth. If your mouth is small, place the dot on the outer ridge of the mouth. If you have a large mouth, the dot should go on the inner ridge of the mouth.

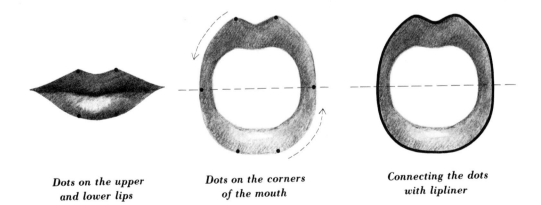

Dots on the upper and lower lips   *Dots on the corners of the mouth*   *Connecting the dots with lipliner*

After the dots of lip color are in place—two on the top lip, two on the bottom lip, and one in each corner of the mouth—connect the dots with a line starting at the center of the mouth and working toward the corners. Do this on both the upper and lower lips.

Now, go back to your lip color, this time putting lots of lipstick on the brush. Using the flat of the brush, fill in the lips with lip color.

These steps may be done entirely with either a lip pencil or lipstick and a lip brush.

When lining your lips, I recommend you choose a lipliner and lipstick that are matched as closely as possible in color. Contrasting lipliners and lipsticks are very artificial-looking. I personally find the look most unattractive. There can be a slight contrast, but it must be very subtle. You might want to use a slightly darker lipliner on a large mouth or full lips to make the mouth appear smaller. Conversely, a slightly lighter lipliner would make a small mouth or thin lips appear fuller.

After the lip color is on your lips, put the lips together and move them gently together, being careful not to smudge the lipline. This pressing together will give a natural balance to the lip color.

If, after pressing your lips together, you think you have too much lipstick on, *very gently* blot the lips with a tissue. Most women put their lipstick on and immediately blot heavily with a tissue—removing most of the lipstick they so carefully put on!

The final step to perfectly made-up lips is lip gloss. The purpose of lip gloss is to create a wet, sexy, voluptuous look. Lip gloss can be very attractive if used properly. However, if lip gloss is applied too heavily and lips end up looking like they are *dripping* color, it becomes very unattractive.

Lip gloss is applied with the lip brush. It should be placed primarily on the lower lip, with just a dab applied on the upper lip. I prefer using a clear, colorless lip gloss. Tinted lip gloss has a tendency to actually change the shade of the lipstick.

You can, however, use a tinted lip gloss as a lipstick. This works best if a lipliner is used first, as the color and consistency of the tinted lip gloss are not definite enough to sustain the lipline. Lip gloss is also a very good way to keep lips from drying out, cracking, and breaking, especially in winter.

Last Steps to Perfect Lips

If, when applying lip color, pressing lips together, or blotting lipstick, you have smudged the lipline, or you need to make some correction on the lips, you can make these corrections with a sponge-tipped or disposable applicator.

Stretch your lips over the teeth, making the lips taut and firm. To correct a smudged lipline, take the applicator and move the smudge up into the lip. The sponge-tipped applicator can also be used to create a perfectly clean, even line by again holding the lips taut over the lips and *cleaning up* any excess lipstick.

After your lips are perfectly made up, smile, and check to make sure that during the application no lip color found its way onto your teeth!

The key to applying lip color perfectly is practice. Keep using a brush or lipliner, resting your pinky on your chin for added control. Keep practicing until, with a lipliner, you can do a perfect touch-up on your lips in a dimly lit restaurant.

To make sure that you get the true shade of lip color each and every time you make up your lips, be sure that your lip brushes are clean. The creamy consistency of lipstick makes it cling to the brush, and color upon color will leave you with brushes of muddy, untrue lipstick shades. Regularly clean your brushes by dipping them in rubbing alcohol, thus allowing them to dry naturally.

7. Finishing Touches to a Perfect Makeup

Once your makeup is completed, it should be *set*, or finished, with translucent powder. This final step of setting the makeup is a step many women skip. It may seem like a small step, but it is the difference between an adequate makeup and a *professional* makeup. It is the small touches in doing a makeup that will produce the finished, porcelain look of a professional makeup. A final dusting with translucent powder will help you achieve that look.

Finishing powders are available in translucent and tinted shades, and in both pressed-powder and loose-powder form. I prefer translucent powder. It achieves the look I want, and the colorlessness of the translucent powder will not change the colors of the makeup already on the face.

Translucent powder is available in a matte finish and in an iridescent form. I recommend you use the matte-finish translucent powder during the day and save the glitter and glow that comes from iridescent powder for the evening.

How to Apply

Translucent powder is applied liberally with the large powder brush. After applying to the entire face—including eyelids and eyelashes—make sure you dust

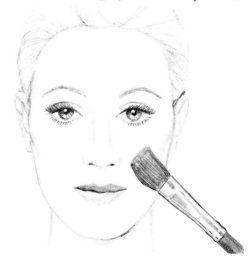

the neck, shoulders, and, if you wish, the cleavage. After applying the powder liberally, make sure you *buff* very vigorously with the powder brush. The soft goat hairs of the powder brush will not irritate your skin, and the vigorous buffing will set the makeup and prevent any loose powder from settling on your clothing.

Translucent powder is particularly important on the eyelashes. It coats the lashes, and when an additional coat of mascara is applied, it will cling to the lashes, making them appear thicker, darker, and longer. Remember to take your eyebrow brush and brush the lashes to remove any excess mascara. Also take a moment to once again reverse the eyebrows with the eyebrow brush and then shape them in the proper direction, making sure brows are free of loose powder.

Translucent Powder for Day and Evening

For daytime, I recommend you use a translucent powder without the iridescence, and use powder more sparingly to avoid a pasty, caked look. A good translucent powder for the daytime should be very sheer.

When the powder is applied properly, it keeps makeup on all day. This is especially helpful for women with oily skin for two reasons: First, the powder will prevent makeup from coming off; and second, it helps prevent the face from getting shiny.

Another way to keep makeup looking great during the day is to be sure you keep a supply of absorbent linen tissues in your makeup bag. Blot the face gently with the tissues to absorb excess oils and perspiration on the face *without* disrupting the makeup.

For the evening, especially when playing to subdued lights, such as restaurant candlelight, use a colorless, iridescent powder. The iridescence will give your makeup a glitter and soft glow that is most attractive in soft light. This works on women of all skin colors with the possible exception of very ebony-skinned black women.

Tinted Powders

Although I prefer translucent powders, there are women who require the extra coverage that tinted powders can give. Women who have excessively ruddy complexions might want a beige-tinted finishing powder to tone down the redness. A woman with an extremely sallow complexion might find that a pink-tinted powder will make her skin tone appear less yellow. Women with problem complexions, such as pockmarks, scars, broken capillaries, etc., might want to use tinted powders as the color will add coverage.

When choosing a tinted powder, make sure that the shade of the tinted powder corresponds to the foundation-base shade. That means if your foundation is in the beige family, your finishing powder, if not translucent, should also be in the beige family.

Women who have good skin but very large pores should stay away from tinted powders. The color tends to accentuate the large pores.

When using tinted powders, it is extremely important to take extra care with buffing the powder to avoid a caked, orangy look. Particular care is required if the powder is to be used around the neck area, because the tinted powders will rub off on clothes and cause discoloration.

Optional Finishing Tips

Setting your makeup with translucent powder will balance your makeup, give it the final blending, and also eliminate any shine from your face. For those of you who want to go one step beyond, here are some tips for the perfectly finished makeup.

1. Take a step back and look at your face in the mirror.
2. Before putting on your translucent powder, apply a white, white-gold, or light beige eye shadow above the cheekbones to highlight and accentuate the tops of the cheekbones.
3. For an evening look, go over the blusher with a light gold or white-gold iridescent eye shadow.
4. Still using the light gold or white iridescent eye shadow *very lightly*, go over all the highlight areas.
5. With a taupe or brown eye shadow, make last-minute contour additions —under the cheekbones, down the sides of the jaw, and under the chin.
6. Dust on translucent or translucent iridescent powder. Buff well with the powder brush.

From the first step in makeup to the last finishing touch, all application is related to the dark/light illusion. This illusion is truly what makeup is all about.

8. Step-by-Step Makeups

The Jerome Alexander Five-Minute Makeup

A question that I'm asked frequently when I appear on television is "What is the one cosmetic you would recommend a woman use, even if she wore absolutely no other makeup?" My answer is that there is no *one* miracle cosmetic—but there are four: foundation, blusher, mascara, and lipstick, which can be applied in five minutes and will allow a woman to enhance her natural looks.

I believe a woman should never walk out of the house without a little makeup on. Although there are some women who have perfect skin, nice natural coloring, and attractively shaped eyes with long, thick, dark lashes, I've seen very few of these natural beauties! Most women need the color and correction a little makeup can provide.

Some women consciously choose not to wear any makeup. They might put on a little mascara, lipstick, and blusher for a very special occasion, but they don't think of makeup as an everyday item. I'm not here to convert the world to makeup. As I've stated repeatedly, women do not want to change the image that they have of themselves. However, if you are reading this book, you probably have more than a passing interest in makeup.

I believe that the majority of women today are spending more money than ever on their appearance. Dollars spent on even casual wardrobes are rising each year. And, of course, more women than ever are working outside the home. Competition in the work force is fierce. Good grooming and an attractive appearance give you a slight edge on the competition. Part of feeling successful in the business world is the ability to know that you look your best.

Although the woman who works outside the home may not have the time (or desire) to spend twenty minutes to one hour each morning applying makeup, *every woman* should develop a five-minute makeup routine.

Let me inject my personal philosophy here. Makeup is not only a face you present to the public, but something you also do for yourself. Often, women who work at home think they have no need for makeup as they are not going to meet anyone during their day. But they are very wrong. Even if your only trip out of the house is to pick up the children at school, you owe it to yourself and your family to look your very best. Children are proud of parents who take time with their appearance. I can remember feeling proud that when my mother came to school she was always nicely dressed and had taken the time to put makeup on. It told me that she cared—about both herself and me.

So, no matter what activities are planned for the day, here is my quick, basic five-minute makeup. In this chapter, I'm only going to give you the steps for the makeups. You learned the how-to for each step in the previous chapters.

1. *Always* use a moisturizer on your face.
2. Apply foundation covering the entire face, eyelids, lips, neck, and ears.
3. Apply a light blusher on the cheekbones. Use a dark contour blusher in the hollow of the cheekbones. Blend well with a sponge wedge.
4. Line the lips with a lipliner pencil. Using a corresponding shade of lipstick, fill in the lips with a lip brush.
5. To give depth and drama to the eyes, apply a coat of mascara to the upper and lower lashes. Separate the lashes by combing through with an eyebrow brush.

The first time you follow these five steps, time yourself. Don't be surprised to find it took less than five minutes for you to put your makeup on! Look at the difference a mere five minutes can make. I'm willing to bet you'll never again use the excuse "I don't have time to put my makeup on!"

The Jerome Alexander Step-by-Step Daytime Makeup

The secret of a good daytime makeup is to get into a pattern without falling into a routine. While writing this book, I spoke to many women who work outside the home and asked them how long it takes them to put their makeup on in the morning. The time ranged from ten minutes to a half-hour. The places where the makeup was applied were as varied as the time it took women to apply makeup. From car pools to makeup tables, from bathrooms to commuter trains. Where you put your makeup on and how long it takes is not crucial. What is important is that you put your makeup on in good light.

What is the right light for applying makeup? Natural daylight is excellent, but unfortunately few people have access to bathrooms with huge skylights. If you are putting your makeup on at home, invest in a makeup mirror that comes with settings to simulate various types of lighting. Most makeup mirrors offer three: daylight, evening light, and office light. Many light-bulb companies are now making bulbs that simulate daylight. You might want to consider replacing the bulbs in your bathroom with these new bulbs.

82

The worst light in which to apply makeup is fluorescent light. It seems to give the skin a greenish tint. Makeup applied under fluorescent light will look very different in natural light or under incandescent light.

In addition to the proper lighting, it is important that you develop a pattern that will allow you to apply your makeup with a minimum of fuss and bother each morning.

Below, I've given you my instruction for a basic daytime makeup. Think of it as a makeup recipe: step by step to a finished product. You may want to follow the recipe the first few times and then experiment until you find a pattern that is tailored to your individual needs. After all, most cooking recipes say "season to taste"!

1. Moisturize your face and neck.
2. Apply foundation.
3. Use concealing cream to cover under-eye shadows.
4. Contour and highlight your face into the illusion of being oval-shaped. For daytime, I recommend using light and dark foundation for the contouring and highlighting. A dark blusher may be used in lieu of a dark foundation.
5. Blusher: Using a dark and light blusher, continue contouring and highlighting the cheekbones.
6. Eyes.
   a. Apply three different eye shadows to the upper eyelid.
   b. Apply a dark eye shadow in the crease of the eyelid.
   c. Highlight the brow bone with a light highlight eye shadow.
   d. Eyeliner can be omitted for a daytime makeup. If you do choose to use an eyeliner, line the upper lid and choose a soft brown liner, avoiding the harsher black eyeliners. Line the platform of the lower lid with a light blue pencil or blue eye shadow.
   e. Apply mascara to the upper and lower lashes. Separate the lashes with a brow brush after the mascara has been applied.
   f. Brush eyebrows into shape. If necessary, lighten or darken brows with a taupe eye shadow.
7. Line the lips with a lipliner pencil. With a corresponding shade of lipstick, fill in the remainder of the lips. For daytime, apply just a slight amount of lip gloss to the lower lip.
8. Finish your daytime makeup by dusting the face with translucent powder. Buff well with the large powder brush.

The Jerome Alexander Complete Evening Makeup

This complete, detailed evening makeup will take from thirty minutes to one hour to apply, depending upon your skill and how much makeup you like to wear. I suggest that evening makeups be practiced many times in advance before the night of a special occasion. The same attention you give to your dress, hair, and accessories should be given to how you will wear your makeup. This is especially true if you are going to experiment and wear your makeup differently than you have in the past.

1. As always, start your makeup by applying a moisturizer to your face and neck.
2. If you have heavy shadows under your eyes, apply concealing cream before you put on your foundation.
3. Foundation should be two shades darker than your actual skin tone. Blend well with a sponge wedge to achieve sheer, even coverage.
4. Contour and highlight your facial shape into the illusion of being oval.
5. Blusher should be two shades: a light, iridescent blusher for the cheekbones; a darker, matte blusher for the hollow of the cheekbones. For an evening look, apply white-gold eye shadow over the light iridescent blusher on top of the cheekbones. The eye shadow will work as an additional highlighter.
6. Eye shadows for evening should be more vibrant than those for daytime. Once again, apply shadows on the upper lid in three parts.
7. Create a definition between the brow bone and the eyelid using a dark, dramatic eye shadow.
8. To highlight the brow bone, choose a very light iridescent eye shadow, such as a white-gold.
9. In the evening, use a darker eyeliner for depth and drama. Both the upper and lower eyelids receive eyeliner. Take care not to ring the eyes with liner as this will make them appear smaller. On the platform of the lower lid, use a vibrant blue pencil or powdered eye shadow.
10. For nighttime, eyelashes should get more than one coat of mascara. After removing the excess mascara by brushing lashes with an eyebrow brush, coat the lashes with a dusting of translucent powder, which helps the mascara cling to lashes. Then apply a second coat of mascara.
11. After shaping the brows with a brow brush, apply some gold eye shadow to your eyebrow brush and brush into the brows.
12. Take a look at your face and make any last-minute adjustments. You can do some final contouring of the nose, cheekbones, jawline, etc., with a taupe eye shadow. A white-gold eye shadow will serve to highlight the tops of the cheeks and also the nose and the chin.
13. The lips should get strong, vibrant lip colors. Pearls and gold-flecked lipsticks are especially popular for evening. After applying lipstick, give the lips a finished evening look by applying lots of clear lip gloss to both the upper and lower lips.
14. This evening makeup is set with lots of iridescent powder to give the makeup a shimmering, glistening look. Make sure to buff briskly with a powder brush.

Whether you are attempting the basic five-minute makeup, the daytime makeup, or the full evening makeup, always remember to follow each step carefully. Practice the entire makeup repeatedly until doing it perfectly becomes second nature.

9. Makeup for Teen-agers

Every year it seems that girls are starting to wear makeup at younger and younger ages. While I can remember my sister, at age sixteen, wiping off her makeup before my father saw her, today it's not at all unusual to see girls thirteen and even younger applying makeup.

One of the reasons for this makeup awareness at a young age is that daughters are learning from their cosmetic-conscious mothers. Most women over thirty have mothers who probably wore only lipstick and blush—maybe mascara and eye shadow for a party. These women learned their makeup savvy from friends, fashion magazines, and trial and error. The young girls of today have grown up with mothers who are beauty- and fitness-conscious. And like all young girls, they want to emulate their mothers.

I'm not going to get into whether it's right or wrong for such young girls to wear makeup. The fact is they are. And a teen-ager can look very pretty wearing cosmetics if she makes herself up like the young girl she is and doesn't try to look like an adult.

Let's look quickly at both the beauty assets and beauty problems of being a teen-ager.

Assets	*Problems*
You have young, tight skin with no wrinkles. To look attractive, teen-agers need very little makeup.	Teen-agers are prone to oily skin and problems such as pimples and blackheads.
The skin has a natural glow. The eyelids are smooth, the lips firm and naturally colored.	Teen-age diets are not known for their nutritional balance. Junk foods contribute to skin problems.

The teen years are an excellent time to get into good beauty routines. Good habits formed now tend to last a lifetime. So if you're a teen-age girl, my advice to you would be to always moisturize your face. Although dry skin and wrinkles are way in the future, *now* is the time to start the battle against aging.

What follows is a basic makeup for teen-agers. For very special occasions, such as the senior prom, you might want to wear a little bit more color. In general, however, I recommend that makeup be kept to a minimum during the teen years. Young, smooth skin and youth's natural coloring are beauty assets that can't be found in a makeup kit.

Foundation. Although some beauty authorities think young girls need not wear foundation, I do not agree. No matter what your age, foundation is the base upon which makeup should rest.

Many teen-age faces have oily skin and should use a water-based foundation. If you are acne-prone, I recommend using a cream foundation, which will provide extra coverage for pimples, pockmarks, and large pores.

If your skin problems become major, now is the time to see a dermatologist. Problem acne should be treated by a physician, not merely concealed with cosmetics.

Foundation is applied with your fingertips and blended with a sponge.

Contouring and Highlighting. Sculpting the face into the illusion of an oval is too dramatic for a young girl's face. However, you can begin practicing the dark/light illusion that you learned about in chapter 2 by using dark and light blushers.

Blusher. Most teen-agers need a minimum of blusher. The natural glow of youth is pretty enough! Blushers should be light pastel shades. Even your darker, contour blusher should not be too dark. Please refer to chapter 3 for the proper way to apply blusher to contour and highlight your cheekbones.

Eyes. For everyday makeup, I would recommend wearing just a *touch* of mascara. When applying mascara, begin by removing the glob that forms at the end of the mascara wand. Hold the wand straight up and move it from side to side across the lashes. This will coat each lash and avoid a clumpy, unnatural look.

If you wish to wear eye shadow, choose neutral colors like taupes, beiges, eggshell, smoky gray, khaki, etc. These colors can contour and highlight the eyes without adding too much color and drama.

Lips. Teen-age lips are usually naturally colored and lipstick is not necessary. I recommend applying a clear gloss to the lips. This will make your naturally rosy lips shine and will provide a young, dewy, wet look. Lip gloss will also protect your lips against chapping and drying.

Eyebrows. Over and over I've said that properly shaped brows are crucial to an attractive face. The shape of your brows sets the expression on your face.

If you start tweezing and shaping your brows properly as a teen-ager, you will have the advantage of a lifetime of beautiful brows.

86

In chapter 5, I've given a step-by-step outline for beautiful brows. Follow it carefully. If you're ever in doubt about whether a hair should be tweezed, my advice is don't tweeze it! Overtweezing at an early age can lead to sparse brows later in life.

I would like to talk a bit about makeup and the teen-age budget. Most teen-agers don't have as much money as they would like to spend on cosmetics, but you shouldn't need to spend a lot for your makeup needs during these years. I would suggest that you invest in a good set of makeup brushes. These are the tools that you need in order to apply your makeup properly.

Also, take care to make your cosmetics and tools last. This means regularly keeping your brushes cleaned, as described in chapter 1.

Your allowance may not cover all the cosmetics you would like to purchase, but, as I said earlier, it is not always necessary to buy the highest-priced products. Many times, inexpensive products will work just as well for you.

My final words to you on makeup: Please avoid sharing your cosmetics with your friends. Although the temptation is to try a friend's mascara or eye shadow, this is an easy way to get eye infections. Keep your cosmetics clean and stored in a cool place, and you'll keep them free of the bacteria that cause eye problems.

10. Makeup for the Mature Woman

When does a woman become a "mature woman"? That's a tough question to answer—and no matter what age I name, I'm sure to make some enemies!

In terms of makeup, most women will begin to notice changes in their facial skin in their thirties; lines may appear that will develop into wrinkles in the forties or fifties and become creases in the sixties and seventies. Of course, these are generalizations and you may pass from decade to decade with smooth, unlined skin.

The ability to look forever young is based upon what I call "the grandmother theory." Take a look at your mother and grandmother— if they have retained a youthful look, chances are good that you have inherited this tendency also.

Age is also more than the face that looks back at you from the mirror. Some women in their late fifties perceive themselves as being young—and they are! They think young, dress young, and act young. And there's not a thing wrong with their attitude. With the right approach to makeup, they can create the illusion of being younger than they actually are.

Other women, at thirty-five years of age, perceive themselves as *mature*. They dress, act, and think of themselves as no longer young. If, during one of my personal appearances, I made up this type of woman to look younger, she would probably not like what she saw in the mirror. Conversely, if I made up a fifty-five-year-old, who perceives herself as young, as a more mature woman, she would also dislike the results. She would most certainly dislike me!

So let me be very clear. As women mature, they develop very definite self-images—which they will fight against changing. Makeup is a very effective way to enhance the woman you are *without* changing your self-perceptions.

Makeup Myths and Mature Women

Women, as they mature, generally assume that they need *more* makeup to look attractive. This is especially true of those women who have always enjoyed wearing makeup. When women begin to see lines, wrinkles, and creases, they feel that

89

extra makeup will provide more coverage. Heavy makeup is counterproductive. Rather than covering flaws, it calls attention to these areas. Women believe that increasing the intensity and depth of color of their makeup will help them look younger. Instead, it gives a harsh, hard effect.

The first lesson for mature women is to lessen the intensity of color, choosing softer, more subtle shades, and to decrease the total amount of makeup applied.

Step-by-Step Makeup Application

All women should moisturize their skin, but for mature women, a moisturizer is crucial. As you get older, the skin loses its ability to retain its natural moisture. I suggest moisturizing as often as possible. Wear moisturizer under makeup and apply a moisturizer when going without makeup as well. Investigate the many extra-rich moisturizers and night creams on the market.

Again, the real secret of a mature woman's makeup is not heavier and more, but lighter and less. Foundation should be sheer and soft. Foundation will *not* cover wrinkles. If you have bad skin, a cream foundation may conceal scars, broken capillaries, pockmarks, etc., but it cannot erase wrinkles.

Use a good concealer (in cream form, liquid, or stick). A shade a bit lighter than your own skin tone is effective for covering shadows under the eyes and can be used as a highlighter for deep wrinkles and creases such as laugh lines between the nose and the mouth. It can also be used on the lines on the forehead caused by frowning and on the crow's feet that appear on the outer corners of the eyes caused by smiling and squinting.

You may be confused by my telling you to highlight the wrinkles. You're probably thinking, I want to make them disappear, not highlight them! It's paradoxical—but true—that by highlighting a wrinkle, you make it seem to disappear, instead of making it seem accentuated, as one would think. A line or crease is actually a shadow on the face. By *highlighting* the shadow, you create the illusion of the shadow (be it a line, wrinkle, or crease) coming forward and blending with the rest of the face to present a smooth appearance.

What I have found to be most effective for the application of concealer is a fine eyeliner brush. This brush allows the concealer to be applied directly in the crease or the line. After application, gently blend with a sponge.

Contouring and Highlighting

Refer to chapter 2 and contour and highlight your natural face shape into an illusion of an oval-shaped face.

As women mature, they tend to develop jowls—excess flesh under the jawline. Shade this area from the end of the chin to the beginning of the jawline.

Also prevalent in older women is a double chin. Shading of this area should start under the jawline and be continued on the chin. Regular contouring and highlighting of the nose, cheeks, forehead, and eyes remain the same regardless of age. Refer to chapter 2 for instructions on contouring and highlighting each facial feature.

Blusher

Dark blushers can be used for contouring, but should be used very sparingly. Light blushers should be chosen from the pastel shades, avoiding the more vibrant colors. Application of blusher remains the same as for younger women (see chapter 3). Just remember to use less and choose lighter colors.

Eyes

What you've learned about dividing the upper eyelid into three parts still applies for the makeup of a mature woman. The difference is, as a woman becomes older, the skin around the eyelids tends to lose its elasticity and take on a crepey look. Gravity takes its toll, too, and heavy upper eyelids are quite common.

Mature women should avoid highly pearlized eye shadows. The iridescence accentuates the crepey skin around the eyes and exaggerates the problem of heavy upper lids. Now is the time to choose lightly pearlized or matte eye shadows.

To reduce the problem of heavy upper lids and create definition between the brow bone and eyelid is the critical step of eye makeup for mature women. This is accomplished with a dark shadow in the crease of the upper eyelid.

Highlighting of the brow bone remains the same, with the mature woman opting for softer pearls.

Dark eyeliner on the upper lid is a makeup step most mature women should omit. The look is too dramatic and too harsh. The real secret of an attractive makeup for mature women is soft, flattering shades. It is also very difficult to get a smooth, even application of eyeliner because of the often wrinkled skin on the upper eyelid. If you must use eyeliner, exchange the dark kohl colors for a medium shade such as blue, green, wine, or light brown. Ideally, mascara should provide enough depth to the eye to eliminate the need for eyeliner.

Eyeliner *will* work on the platform of the lower lid when you line this area with a blue pencil. This works on women of all ages to make the eyes appear larger and the whites of the eyes seem brighter.

Finish the eye makeup with mascara. I recommend a soft shade like brown or off-black, rather than harsh, blue-black mascara. Apply mascara as detailed in chapter 4, making sure to coat every lash. I've noticed that as some women age, they tend to lose eyelashes and their lashes become very sparse. To give the illusion of thicker and more plentiful lashes, between coats of mascara, powder lashes with translucent powder. After each application of mascara, separate lashes with a brow brush to remove excess mascara.

Eyebrows

As a woman matures, her eyebrows start to become wiry from many years of continuous tweezing and shaping. This does not mean she should cease shaping her brows now! It is important to keep brows well trimmed and shaped, the way I explained in chapter 5.

Even if eyebrows are missing from years of overtweezing, I do not recommend filling in the missing brow with pencil. Instead, use a nylon-tipped eyebrow brush, choosing a neutral eye shadow like taupe, and create the brow with natural, feathery strokes. If your hair has become gray, choose a charcoal-gray eye shadow. Be careful to keep the color very subtle and soft.

Lips

For mature women, one of the most common makeup problems is applying lipstick properly. As the skin ages, creases, wrinkles, smile lines, etc., form around the mouth. If lipstick is applied directly from the stick, the color will bleed into these lines, creating an unattractive, messy look. By lining the lips with a lipliner pencil, which contains extra paraffin (wax) and then filling in lips with a corresponding color, the color will remain inside the lipline (see chapter 6 for application details). Be sure not to go over the lipliner with lipstick or you will lose the effects of the paraffin in the lipliner.

Mature women should choose lighter shades of lipstick and avoid very highly pearlized colors—they are just too flashy. Even women with large mouths, who at an earlier age I recommend use dark lip colors, should now opt for lighter shades. Lip gloss should be used very sparingly. The wet look works well on young women, but it is inappropriate for the more mature woman.

Powder

The setting of makeup with translucent powder is the most important final step. In the evening, translucent, iridescent powder gives a soft, flattering look to mature women. For daytime, use a plain translucent powder. Be sure to powder the entire face and include the neck, ears, and shoulders. Buff well with a large powder brush.

Plastic Surgery

As a woman gets older, she begins to lose the muscle tone she had when younger. Like the muscles found elsewhere in the body, the facial muscles, when not exercised, become slack. This loss of muscle tone, combined with the natural force of gravity, causes the face to sag.

Many women think the answer to this problem is plastic surgery. Once operations were for the very rich and the very famous, today women from all walks of life are having elective cosmetic surgery. I personally believe in plastic surgery, though I know not all women can afford it, nor are all women psychologically prepared for it.

One operation that I have seen incredible results from is the removal of the bags under the eyes caused by fatty tissue deposits. These fatty deposits are already noticeable in the early twenties and can be removed as soon as they are noticeable. Once removed, they generally do not recur. Operations to correct heavy upper eyelids also take years off a woman's apparent age.

If you are considering plastic surgery, here are some points to consider.

- Above all, chose a reputable surgeon. Call the local board of plastic surgeons or the American Medical Association to recommend a physician in your area.
- Speak with friends who have undergone plastic surgery. Critically examine their results.
- When visiting the doctor's office, insist on seeing *patients*, not pictures, to evaluate his or her skills.
- Don't be afraid to ask the surgeon all your questions. Many women feel intimidated in a physician's office, and end up asking their questions of their friends instead of the doctor. Make sure you ask about the cost of the procedure, any risks in the surgery, how long the recuperation process is, and whether the surgery is necessary just once or will need to be repeated five, ten, or fifteen years later. You might find it helpful to jot down your questions as they occur to you. Take your list of questions with you when you visit the doctor, making note of the doctor's answers.
- Be realistic in your expectations. Plastic surgery can change the way you look. It will not change *you* the person. Examine your reasons for wanting the surgery.

Let me close by saying that an attractive woman in her forties, fifties, or sixties can be as beautiful as a pretty twenty-year-old—and certainly more interesting. Mature women really want to get rid of the surface lines and wrinkles, but not the decades and life experiences that produced them.

One of my favorite questions to ask when making up a mature woman is "Would you like to look twenty years younger?" Practically all women answer *no*. Their goal is to look terrific in *their* age group. This goal is easily attained through good exercise, skin care, and the magic of makeup.

11. Makeup for Ethnic Women

In this chapter, I will be talking about the special makeup needs of the black, Hispanic, and Oriental woman. Although the principles of makeup, such as the dark/light illusion, are identical for black, Hispanic, Oriental, and Caucasian women, certain features of the black, Hispanic, and Oriental face need to be made up differently for maximum beauty.

I would like to make it very clear that the suggestions and descriptions that I will be discussing are not meant to be taken as a routine, never to be altered. In particular, the descriptions of the diagrams on the color photos describe colors that are right for those individual models. When following the instructions, keep to the same dark/light—illusion principles, while choosing shades most flattering to your individual skin tone and facial features.

Makeup for the Oriental Woman

Oriental women are among the most exotic beauties in the world. With the proper application of makeup, the results can be stunning.

Foundation

The complexion of the Oriental woman is generally sallow. As you learned in chapter 1, a sallow complexion can be balanced to a neutral beigeness by a pink foundation.

Apply the foundation to the face with your fingertips. Place dots of foundation on the forehead, cheeks, chin, nose, jaw, and neck. Include foundation on the eyelids, ears, and lips.

Using a sponge wedge, blend the foundation in upward strokes until a sheer beige tone appears, replacing the Oriental sallowness.

Contouring and Highlighting

Oriental women also contour and highlight the face into the illusion of being oval-shaped. Anything that falls outside the oval should be contoured with a dark shade. Areas of the face that fall inside will be highlighted with light cosmetics.

The Oriental woman should pay particular attention to her nose when contouring and highlighting her face. Many Oriental women have broad noses. To diminish the width of the nose and create the illusion of a slimmer nose, shade down the sides of the nose beginning almost at the bridge of the nose. Shade the tip of the nose. Highlight down the center of the nose.

Blusher

The principle of blusher—light blusher highlighting the cheekbones, and darker blusher contouring the hollows of the cheek—remains the same.

Eyes

The eyes of an Oriental woman are distinctly different from those of a Caucasian, black, or Hispanic woman. When the eyes are open, the eyelid seems to disappear. From what you've already learned, you know that when the eye is open and you cannot see an eyelid, a woman is said to have heavy upper lids. Although Caucasian, black, and Hispanic women can have heavy upper lids (and frequently do develop them as they mature), Oriental women almost *always* have eyes that, when open, do not reveal the eyelids.

To give the illusion of an eyelid being visible when the eye is open, it is necessary to create definition between the brow bone and the upper eyelid. Beginning at the corner of the eye closest to the nose and continuing to the end of the eyelid, apply a dark contour shadow in the crease of the eye. To find the crease of the eye, gently run your finger over the eyelid. The crease is the indentation between the brow bone and the eyelid. On other eyes, the line should remain in the crease, but Oriental eyes need added definition, so the line should be thicker and fall slightly on the brow bone and slightly on the eyelid.

Because of the minimal eyelid, Oriental eyes can appear to be less concave and convex than other eyes. To make eyes appear less flat, and take on added depth, apply eyeliner to the natural shape of the eyes. The dark liner will make lashes appear thicker and give depth to the eyes.

The rest of the makeup for the Oriental eye follows the same principles as those for the Caucasian woman. The upper eyelid should receive a dark shadow on the last one-third of the lid, a light highlight shade in the center of the lid, and a light shade on the first third of the lid if the eyes are close-set and a dark eye shadow if eyes are widely spaced. Evenly spaced eyes can choose either a light or dark shade of eye shadow for the first one-third of the upper eyelid.

Finish eyes by applying mascara as you learned in chapter 4. Make sure eyebrows are properly shaped and tweezed. Oriental women have hair that ranges from the darkest brown to black. If the eyebrows need to be darkened, instead of using a dark grease pencil, take an eyebrow brush and gently, with feathery strokes, brush in a dark brown eye shadow.

Lips

There are no special instructions for lip-color application for the Oriental woman. Like her Caucasian counterpart, she should make up her lips to create the illusion that they are evenly shaped. Look in the mirror to determine what type of lips you have, then refer to the instructions in chapter 6 to properly make up your lips.

Finishing Touches

Dust the face with translucent powder for daytime, iridescent powder for night. Apply powder liberally with a large powder brush to the face, neck, and shoulders. Buff well with the powder brush to remove excess powder and set the makeup.

I recommend using a colorless powder. If you do use a tinted powder, be sure to use a pink tinted powder to complement the pink-based foundation you applied to combat the natural sallowness of Oriental skin.

Makeup for the Black Woman

The complexions of black women range from the lightest coffee color to the deepest ebony. Recognizing that all black women do not have the same skin coloring, I will be discussing makeup needs of the black woman in terms of individual features, rather than focusing on complexions.

Many cosmetic companies have lines designed specifically for black women. Black women, however, need not limit their purchases to these cosmetics, be-cause, *with the exception of foundation, there is no difference in the cosmetic color needs of black and Caucasian women.* Black women may choose deeper, more vibrant shades of makeup, but these can be found within most makeup product lines.

Foundation

Of all makeup products, foundation is the one cosmetic that black women should choose differently than other ethnic groups. While Caucasian women choose foundation to achieve an overall beige tone, and Oriental women choose pink foundations to balance their natural sallowness, black women need to match their foundation as closely as possible to their natural skin tone.

Foundations made for black skin are still usually not an exact match to the many different hues of black skin. Most black women will need to purchase two or more shades of foundation and then blend an individual shade that matches their skin tone. Black women should choose the same shade of foundation for both day and evening makeups. Because of the natural coloring of the skin, there is no need to use a foundation two shades darker than your natural skin coloring for evening makeup.

Some black women have uneven skin coloring. There may be a noticeable difference of color on the face. Choose the foundation that most closely matches the darker skin color. If you have oily skin, choose a water-based foundation. If your skin tends to be dry, you should use an oil-based foundation. Sometimes ebony-skinned women with dry skin find their skin taking on an ashen look. This can be corrected by using a moisturizing cream. Of course, no matter what your skin type or coloring, every woman should apply moisturizer to her face before putting on makeup foundation.

Contouring and Highlighting

Makeup for black women, as for all women, works on the principle of the dark/light illusion. Even very dark-skinned women are able to contour and highlight their faces into the illusion of being oval-shaped. The secret of contouring and highlighting for black women is to choose a light brown or beige color for highlighting and a deeper brown shade for contouring. How light (or dark) a highlight shade you choose depends upon your individual skin color.

With your contour and highlight cosmetics, you will contour any part of your face that falls outside an oval shape, and highlight areas of the face that fall inside the oval.

Many black women have noses that range from medium-broad to almost flat. To diminish the width of the nose and create the illusion of a slimmer nose, shade down the sides of the nose and highlight down the center of the nose. Shade the tip of the nose. Where you begin shading the nose depends upon its width. An almost flat nose needs to be shaded starting almost at the bridge of the nose. In chapter 2, you will find detailed instructions and illustrations for contouring and highlighting your nose.

Blusher

Black women should apply blusher as you learned in chapter 3. A highlight blusher is applied to the cheekbones, and a darker blusher contours the hollows under the cheekbones. Dark skin can wear deeper, more vibrant colors. Shades such as plums, burgundies, and bronzes as dark blushers are especially flattering to black skin. The light blusher should be one of the vibrant shades.

Eyes

Everything you learned about making up your eyes, as described in chapter 4, pertains to black women. Remember to apply shadow on the upper eyelid in three parts: The first third of the eyelid gets a light shadow if your eyes are close-set, and a dark shadow if your eyes are wide-set; the center of the eyelid receives a highlight shadow; the last third of the eyelid gets a dark shadow.

Again, darker skin offers the option of choosing bright, vibrant eye shadows. Pearlescent and metallic golds, bronzes, and coppers can be very dramatic.

When the platform of the lower lid is lined with a light blue pencil, the whites of the eyes become even whiter, giving the eyes an extra-large, dramatic appearance.

Lips

Determine your lip shape as you learned in chapter 2 and make up your lips to give them the appearance of being evenly shaped. Some black women have large, sensual mouths with full, voluptuous lips. You should line your lips beginning on the inner ridge with a dark lipliner. When you apply dots to the corners of the mouth, as you learned in chapter 6, make sure the dots are again on the inner ridge of the mouth. Fill in the lips with a dark, corresponding shade of lipstick to minimize their fullness. Avoid light shades and pearlescent lip colors as they will make your mouth look larger and your lips appear fuller.

Finishing Touches

Dust the face with translucent powder for daytime; iridescent powder for night. Apply powder liberally with a large powder brush to the face, neck, and shoulders. Buff well with the powder brush to remove excess powder and set makeup. I recommend using a colorless powder. If you do use a tinted powder, be sure to mix several powders until you have a shade that matches your foundation.

Tinted powders are available that enable a woman to do her makeup with one product. These powders are made from natural clays and minerals. When brushed on the face, they react with the body's own chemistry to produce a warm, glowing look. The powder performs the duty of contour, blusher, eye shadow, and even lip color. These powders work exceptionally well on black skin, bringing a warm, overall glow to the face.

Makeup for the Hispanic Woman

The skin tone, hair coloring, and eye colors of Hispanic women vary greatly. I have known blue-eyed, blond Hispanic women as well as dark-skinned, black-eyed women of Hispanic descent. In this section, I will be talking about the makeup needs of Hispanic women who are dark-skinned with brunette hair and dark eyes.

Dark-skinned Hispanic women tend to have sallow complexions. These women should choose pink-based foundations to balance their skin tone to a more neutral beigeness. Dark Hispanic skin tones range from a deep olive to a dark brown. Many Hispanic women, like black women, will find it necessary to mix several foundation shades until they achieve the shade that is right for their skin tone. My advice to you, for both day and evening makeup, is to match your foundation as closely as possible to your natural skin tone.

Hispanic women who are brunettes with dark skin and dark eyes can wear vibrant, bright shades of makeup. Eye shadows can be extra deep, as can your dark blushers. The deeper skin tone allows you to be flattered by metallic and pearlescent cosmetics.

Excess facial hair, especially above the upper lip, can be a problem for Hispanic women. You don't actually have more hair above the lip than other ethnic groups, but because it tends to be dark hair, it casts a shadow and appears more noticeable.

There are many ways to remove this hair. Waxing and depilatory creams will remove the surface hair. Because the follicle of the hair remains, it will eventually grow back. Waxes and depilatories are sold over the counter at drugstores and are an at-home, do-it-yourself process.

Bleaches are also available, which will not remove the hair but will lighten it to the point where it becomes almost unnoticeable.

Electrolysis is the only way to permanently remove facial hair. This method uses an electrical impulse to actually kill the root of the hair follicle, thereby preventing the hair from regrowing. *This procedure must be performed by a licensed electrologist.* While electrolysis is more expensive than creams, bleaches, and waxes, it is the only way to rid yourself permanently of unwanted hair.

For a truly dramatic look to your eyes, I suggest that Hispanic women, in addition to wearing vibrant eye shadows, line the upper and lower eyelids with a dark eyeliner. Blend the liner carefully and smudge in an upward motion toward the brow bone for a truly exotic look.

Every makeup lesson you have learned in this book applies to Hispanic women. Study your features carefully and make yourself up according to the dark/light principle that is the basis of all makeup.

100

Four Perfect Makeups

Makeup for the Caucasian woman

1 or 2

4

13

12

8 7 6

9

10

3

2 10 11

1

2

4

1 or 2

1 or 5

2

14

Key

Contour
Highlight
Under-eye concealer
Light blusher
Dark, contour blusher
Light eye shadow for close-set eyes, dark eye shadow for wide-set eyes, dark or light eye shadow for evenly spaced eyes
Highlight eye shadow on the center of the upper eyelid
Dark eye shadow for the outer third of the upper eyelid
Eye contour in the crease of the eye socket
Eyeliner on the upper and lower eyelids
Lining the platform of the lower eyelid with a light blue pencil
Highlight on the brow bone
Properly shaped eyebrows
Lip color

4

1 or 2

1 or 2

Note: Where the key shows a choice of a contour (1) or highlight (2) cosmetic, choose the cosmetic that will give your features the illusion of being ideally shaped.

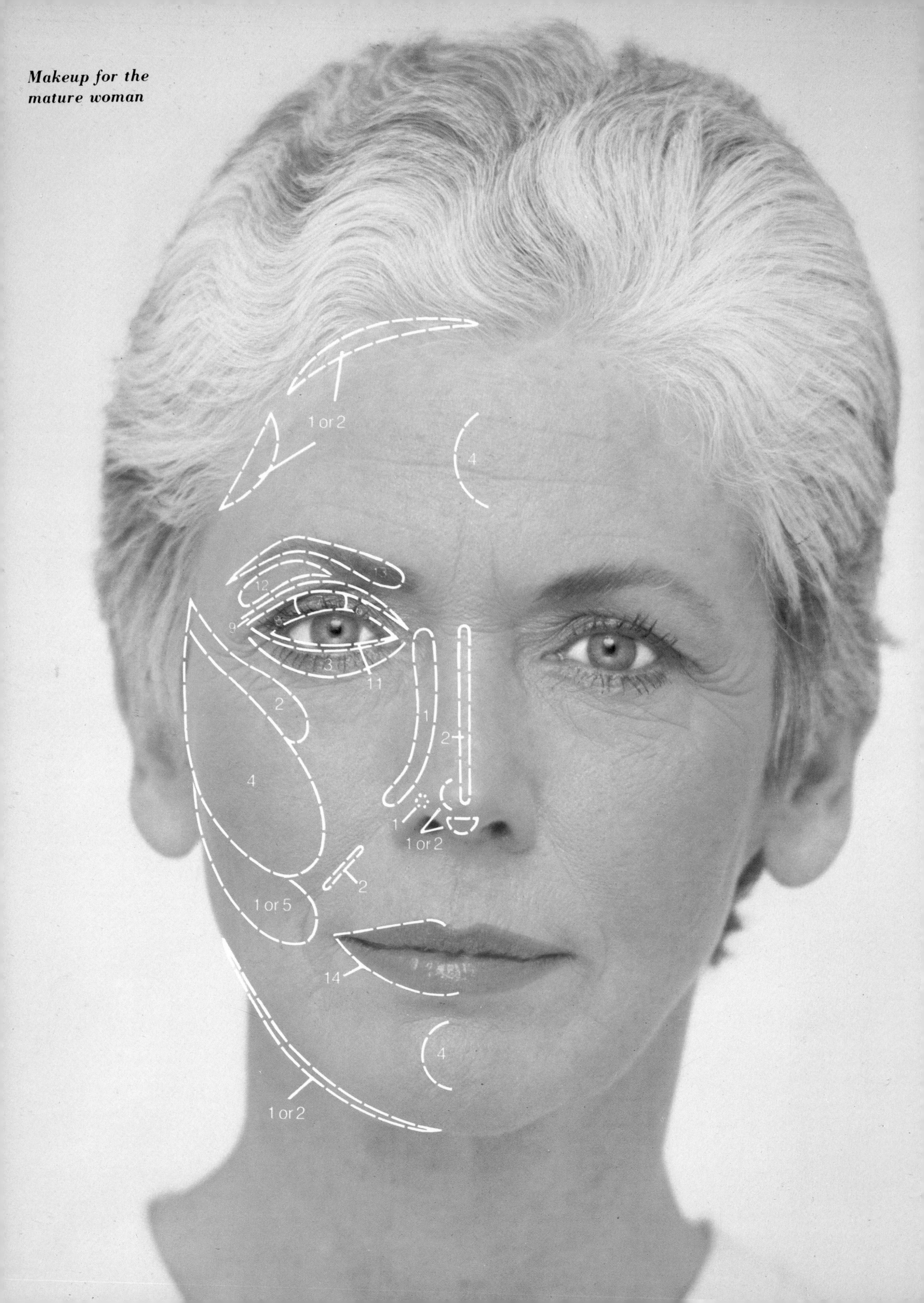

1 or 2
4
13
12
8
9
3
11
2
1
2
4
1
1 or 2
2
1 or 5
14
4
1 or 2

Makeup for the black woman

Key

1 Contour
2 Highlight
3 Under-eye concealer
4 Light blusher
5 Dark, contour blusher
6 Light eye shadow for close-set eyes, dark eye shadow for wide-set eyes, dark or light eye shadow for evenly spaced eyes
7 Highlight eye shadow on the center of the upper eyelid
8 Dark eye shadow for the outer third of the upper eyelid
9 Eye contour in the crease of the eye socket
10 Eyeliner on the upper and lower eyelids
11 Lining the platform of the lower eyelid with a light blue pencil
12 Highlight on the brow bone
13 Properly shaped eyebrows
14 Lip color

Note: Where the key shows a choice of a contour (1) or highlight (2) cosmetic, choose the cosmetic that will give your features the illusion of being ideally shaped.

Makeup for the Oriental woman

1 or 2

4

13

12

9

7

6

8

10

10 11 3

1

2

2

1

1 or 2

2

14

1 or 5

4

1 or 2

4

Key

1 Contour
2 Highlight
3 Under-eye concealer
4 Light blusher
5 Dark, contour blusher
6 Light eye shadow for close-set eyes, dark eye shadow for wide-set eyes, dark or light eye shadow for evenly spaced eyes
7 Highlight eye shadow on the center of the upper eyelid
8 Dark eye shadow for the outer third of the upper eyelid
9 Eye contour in the crease of the eye socket
10 Eyeliner on the upper and lower eyelids
11 Lining the platform of the lower eyelid with a light blue pencil
12 Highlight on the brow bone
13 Properly shaped eyebrows
14 Lip color

Note: Where the key shows a choice of a contour (1) or highlight (2) cosmetic, choose the cosmetic that will give your features the illusion of being ideally shaped.

12. Looking Beautiful When . . .

Makeup and Wearing Eyeglasses

It was Dorothy Parker who said, "Men don't make passes at girls who wear glasses." That statement could not be further from the truth! Today, glasses are a fashion accessory for many beautiful women. The diverse choice of frames and lens tints offers the most flattering pair of eyeglasses for all women.

For women who need prescription lenses, glasses are, in fact, a beauty tool! If you think I'm exaggerating the virtue of glasses, consider these facts. Women who should wear glasses and don't, thinking they'll make them unattractive, end up squinting to see. Squinting is a major cause of crow's feet and furrows in the brow. Tired eyes become red—certainly not an attractive feature. And, finally, the strain of using your eyes without your glasses can cause headaches. It's a simple truth that you can't look good if you don't feel good. So, the next time you reach for your glasses, think of them as the aid that protects your beautiful eyes —much the same way you apply moisturizing cream to protect your skin.

One of the questions I'm most often asked at my beauty seminars is "How do I wear my makeup if I wear glasses?" Application of makeup is really not that different. One of the key steps of a beautiful makeup for women who wear glasses is to make sure you have the right-shaped frames for your face. No matter how skillfully you apply your makeup, the wrong frames will give your face a distorted, unbalanced look.

Below, I've given guidelines for the proper type frames for the different face shapes. Remember, when you look for frames, there is not just one rectangular frame or square frame. Keep in mind the size of your face and choose frames accordingly.

Oval face. The oval face is the ideally shaped face and can choose any style frame.

Round face. The face will appear less round when wearing glasses with more defined angles. Geometric shapes such as square frames look well on a round face.

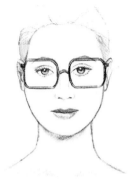

Inverted triangle. Because the inverted-triangle face is widest at the forehead, eyeglass frames that are heavier on the bottom will balance out the disproportion of the face.

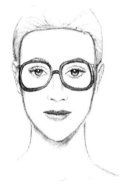

Triangle. The opposite of the inverted triangle, in this case the forehead is the narrowest part of the face. Broad-rimmed frames will give added width to the top portion of the face.

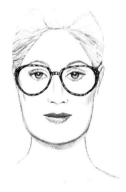

Square. This face shape needs frames with soft, curving lines to diminish the straight lines of the square face.

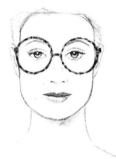

Oblong. Since the oblong face is longer than it is wide, the illusion of additional width can be provided by eyeglass frames that are extra wide.

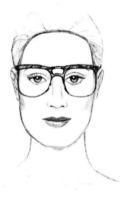

Diamond. The diamond face is all angles, narrowest at the forehead and chin, widest across the face. Try frames with soft, curving lines. Avoid extra-wide frames.

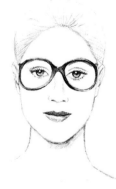

The following chart explains the effects eyeglasses will have on the appearance of your eyes and eye makeup, and also explains the correct way to make up your eyes.

Farsighted lenses magnify eyes and makeup.	Cut down on the amount of eye makeup you use and opt for neutral and beige eye shadows.
Nearsighted lenses minimize eyes.	Eyeliner on the top and lower eyelids brings depth and drama to the eyes.
Bifocals both magnify and distort the appearance of the eye area.	Women who wear bifocals should use soft, subtle shades and a minimum of eye makeup. Bifocals are usually worn by more mature women, who, even if they don't wear glasses, should be applying less makeup.
Glasses call attention to dark shadows under the eyes.	Use a good concealing cream both under foundation and again after the application of foundation.
Glasses can make eyes appear to be close-set.	On the inner corner of the eye, apply a light highlight eye shadow to give the illusion of eyes being evenly spaced.
Tinted lenses can cause a change in the appearance of eye-shadow colors.	Neutral shadows work best with tinted lenses. Avoid lenses and shadows that clash, such as pink lenses and bright green eye shadow.
Eyeglasses that fall below the brow will give a surprised look to the face.	Select frames that rest directly on top of the eyebrows. Trim and shape brows as you normally would.
Strong prescription lenses for farsightedness will magnify eyes and any surrounding wrinkles.	Choose small frames that do not extend beyond the immediate eye area.
Eyeglasses tend to diminish the convex and concave appearance of the eye area, which causes the area to appear flat.	Wear enough dark mascara to give eyes the depth that glasses can take away.

Clear eyeglasses that are extra thick or have an apparent bifocal line will draw attention away from eye makeup.

Have tinted lenses put in the frames. The tint can hide the thickness and the bifocal line.

The wrong frame color on your glasses will prevent a totally pulled-together look.

Keep in mind your natural coloring. Frames should not clash with hair and skin coloring—too many different colors are distracting. Younger women can wear bold red frames, but more mature women should select pale frames.

Tinted glasses can give a tinted cast to the entire eye.

To emphasize the whites of the eye, rim the platform of the lower lid with a blue pencil.

Glasses should not cover the cheek area, as they will cover too much of your face and inhibit the effects of blusher.

Make sure glasses don't extend to where blush should be. When applying blush, put glasses on first.

Glasses can make the face appear top-heavy.

Always wear lipstick when wearing glasses—even if it's the only makeup you have on. Color on the lips will balance the face.

Because glasses today are more than just an aid for eyes, you should have several pairs to complement your wardrobe for different occasions. An eyeglass wardrobe should include a neutral frame that will complement your working wardrobe; a more exotic frame for evenings; a shatterproof frame and shatterproof lenses for sports activities; a pair of sunglasses. Sunglasses should be mandatory for all. Even women who do not wear prescription glasses need the protection sunglasses offer.

Contact Lenses

Contact lenses are an exciting alternative for the times when you don't want to wear glasses. Available in hard and soft lenses, presently only the hard lenses can be tinted, and they will actually change the color of your eyes!

Makeup for contact-lens wearers does not differ from that of women who don't wear glasses. If you do wear lenses, here are some tips on your makeup application to assure that eyes do not become irritated.

- I prefer that you put your contact lenses in after you have applied your eye makeup. However, sometimes eyes tear when lenses are inserted, which will make it necessary to remove eye makeup and begin again! If this frequently happens to you, you will probably want to put lenses in before starting your makeup.
- Avoid waterproof mascaras. Mascara particles sometimes find their way into the eye. Water-soluble mascaras can be flushed out easily with less chance of irritation.
- When lining the platform of the lower lid with a blue pencil, take care if you leave the contact lens in not to have the lens shift or fall out.
- Remove contact lenses before you begin to take off makeup. Even gentle rubbing around the eye area may be uncomfortable if lenses are in the eyes.

Beauty During Pregnancy*

Much has been written about the special glow of pregnancy. Many men find pregnant women especially beautiful, yet many women who are pregnant don't feel beautiful at all! It is possible to go from the first weeks of pregnancy until the delivery day both looking and feeling beautiful.

I know that beauty is possible during pregnancy not just from the viewpoint of a professional makeup artist but from personal experience within my own family. When my wife of fifteen years, Geraldine, was pregnant with our son, Berin James, she never looked less than her absolute best. Although her body, skin, and hair underwent the normal changes of pregnancy, by adapting her makeup routines to these changes she always looked sensational. *And so can you!*

Psychologically, I feel it is imperative that a woman feel beautiful during pregnancy. This is especially true of first-time mothers. Uncertainty, nervousness, and some lack of confidence are all a normal part of the nine months preceding parenthood. Knowing you look your best will help you feel better and stronger.

The reasons your body, skin, and hair undergo changes during pregnancy are hormones. At the end of the first trimester of pregnancy, almost eighteen pregnancy-related hormones are present. Many of these hormones can turn out to be beauty assets. If you are feeling a bit queasy in the mornings, take heart from the following facts.

- If you are acne-prone, pregnancy can clear up this condition! In many cases, your clear skin will remain after you've had your baby!
- Your hair may feel its thickest and look its most luxurious during pregnancy. This is because, although hair is constantly shedding and regrowing, during pregnancy the shedding phase comes to almost a complete standstill. The truth is, you simply have more hair on your head!

*The situations discussed in this chapter may or may not arise during a pregnancy. Any conditions that occur during your pregnancy should be discussed with your obstetrician.

• Nails, too, seem to become stronger and grow at a more rapid rate. Women who never had strong nails prior to being pregnant notice that beautiful nails are an unexpected bonus of having a baby. These longer nails will help your hands look slimmer if they tend to puff up with added weight.

Of course, there are also conditions of pregnancy that are not as desirable to overall beauty. They are, however, easily correctable with makeup.

Oily skin. Some women experience excessively oily skin during pregnancy. I suggest you use a water-based foundation during this time. Also, you might want to use a skin freshener with a higher alcohol content than the one you were using.

Dry skin. For some women, excessively dry skin may be the problem during pregnancy. Moisturizing creams are the best treatment for dry skin. You might want to invest in a super-rich night cream and moisturize your face before bedtime. If dry skin is your problem, choose an oil-based foundation to wear under your makeup.

Mask of pregnancy. You might notice brown or yellow skin discolorations that appear on the face and neck. Degrees of discoloration may vary, but the condition usually goes away a short time after delivery. Brunettes and dark-skinned women seem to be the most susceptible to this "mask of pregnancy."

To correct this condition with makeup, use a concealing cream—the same cream you use to cover under-eye shadows. With your fingers, pat a small amount over the areas to be covered. Blend well with a sponge. Apply your makeup foundation over the concealer. This should cover most discolorations. If some dark spots can still be seen through the foundation, apply additional concealer over your base foundation. Make sure to blend well. Both foundation and concealer should match your own skin tone for day makeup and should be one to two shades darker for evening makeup.

Fuller face. During pregnancy, your face will probably become fuller. It is next to impossible to gain the weight necessary to have a healthy baby and not have some weight gain in the face. Water retention can also account for the appearance of a fuller face.

Does this mean you have to abandon the illusion of an oval-shaped face? Not at all! It may be a fuller oval, but the illusion is still possible with properly applied makeup.

The additional weight in your face may make a usually square face appear round; an inverted triangle seem square; etc. So, disregard what you know to be your true face when contouring and highlighting. Instead, look in the mirror and reexamine your face shape. The same dark/light principle of makeup applies when you are pregnant. With your hands, make an oval around your face. As always, anything that falls outside the oval should be contoured to make it appear smaller, and anything that falls inside the oval should be highlighted to make it appear larger and seem to come forward. You might find that now you are doing a lot more contouring than you did before!

Be sure to repeat the motion of making the oval with your hands around your face as you advance through your pregnancy, since your face will continue to change.

The rest of your makeup should be applied as you usually apply it. You might find you need a little less highlight blusher on the cheekbones, forehead, tip of the chin, and tip of the nose. The beautiful glow of pregnancy often colors these areas naturally. Do, however, make sure to apply your contour blusher in the hollow of your cheekbones. Your new, fuller face needs this definition.

Looking Beautiful in the Hospital

Many women, especially first-time mothers, are shocked to find that they haven't lost all their extra weight the day the baby is born. This shouldn't come as that much of a surprise, because although a thirty-pound weight gain is quite normal during a pregnancy, thirty-pound babies are very rare! Your figure will come back with a little discipline on your part. There is no reason, however, why you can't look and feel pretty when you receive your first visitors in the hospital after the baby is born. All it takes is a little planning.

Before you are scheduled to deliver, treat yourself to a day of professional beauty care. I don't recommend that you wait until the last minute for these appointments. Babies have been known to arrive ahead of schedule!

- Have a professional facial.
- Visit your hairdresser. Get a trim or try a new style. If you are trying something new, insist on an easy-maintenance style that will require little upkeep during the baby's first weeks.
- Get your legs waxed to remove excess hair.
- Have a manicure and pedicure. Remember that the nail polish may be removed by the hospital staff prior to delivery, so be sure to pack some nail polish in your hospital bag.

You will be amazed at how much better you'll feel when you're on the way to the hospital. One woman, when asked about the delivery of her third child, remembers being embarrassed because it was the only time she gave birth when she hadn't shaved her legs!

When you pack the bag for the hospital, make sure your makeup bag is included among the layette and disposable diapers. Be sure to include a makeup mirror, preferably one with different light settings. Hospitals are often green-walled with fluorescent lighting. Not the best light for applying makeup!

After the Baby is Born . . .

"I'm just trying to cope!" are words most often expressed by new mothers. Lack of sleep, lack of energy, a total devotion to the baby are the reasons most often given for not looking their very best. "Who has the time?" is a frequent complaint. "*You* have the time," is my answer! Not only the time but the right to indulge the wish to be beautiful. The Jerome Alexander Five-Minute Makeup, described in chapter 8, is the answer to your time-pressed day. Every new mother has five minutes to devote to herself. Let your husband change the diaper while you put on your makeup. And if he's not used to the diaper routine, you'll get more than five minutes!

Set beauty time aside while your baby naps. Newborns generally sleep most of the time—although it may not seem that way! While the baby naps, take time for a manicure, at-home facial, or pedicure.

Above all, accept the fact that through your pregnancy, during your hospital stay, and while you are at home with your baby, you deserve to look your very best.

Beauty and the Sun

The sun, the sea, the sand. All the elements that make for glorious summer days are the natural enemies of a beautiful you. Every year more research brings alarming news about the sun. Its ultraviolet rays, taken too frequently and for prolonged periods of time, can be hazardous to both your health and your good-looks.

Still, most fashion magazines show bronzed beauties enjoying the pleasures of the beach, and most women take out the tanning oil at the first sign of summer. Personally, I am a sun lover and know I look better when my skin is tanned. However, knowing the damage that the sun can do to the skin, I take precautions to get a *healthy* glow. If you follow my directions for summer beauty, you will find that it is possible to be beautiful on the beach while taking in the sun.

- *Always tan gradually!* This means choosing a suntan lotion with the highest sun block—known as Skin Protection Factor (SPF)—for your first days out. Limit your tanning time to a half-hour until you get a base of color.
- *Skin-protection factors are numbered 2–15.* An SPF of 2 offers the least protection from the sun's ultraviolet rays and is used only after you've got a good base tan. The "2" stands for twice the protection you get sunbathing without suntan lotion. The sun protection factor increases up to an SPF of 15, which acts almost as a complete sun block. Gradually decrease the SPF of your tanning lotion, and increase the amount of time you spend in the sun.
- *Know your skin type!* Generally, olive-skinned brunettes tan easily, while fair-skinned redheads tend to burn. However, the ability to tan is based upon how much melanin (skin pigment) your body produces when exposed to the sun. So, you may be a blonde who tans easily, or a brunette who burns. If the sun is not your ally, don't try to battle it! You can simulate the appearance of a tan with cosmetics. There are powders made of natural clays and minerals that, when brushed on the skin, react with your own body chemistry to give a glowing,

bronzed look to your face. They are totally natural-looking and you'll have the beauty of a tan without the damage excess sun can cause.

- *Moisturize! Moisturize!* Moisturizing your skin is important all year round, but when you're out in the sun, it is especially crucial. While the sun is tanning your skin, it is also stripping the body of water. This dehydration of the skin's natural water supply is what gives the leathery look to the skin and the feeling of tightness. Moisturizers will restore the water and lubricate the skin. They will also help prevent or forestall the peeling process, which begins when the skin sheds cells that have been tanned too quickly.

In addition to enjoying the sun safely and sensibly, these are the beauty items I recommend you bring along for a day at the beach:

Sun glasses
Plant mister filled with mineral
   water
Waterproof cosmetic bag
Foot cream
Beach hat made of natural fiber
Moisturizer
Lemons

Sun glasses. In addition to protecting your eyes from the sun's ultraviolet rays, sunglasses will prevent you from squinting—one of the major causes of wrinkles on the forehead and crow's feet around the eyes.

Beach hat made of natural fiber. A large cotton straw hat will help prevent heatstroke. In addition, the natural fiber will let your hair breathe. Perspiration is as big an enemy as sun to color-treated hair.

Plant mister filled with mineral water. This has many beauty uses on the beach. After coming out of the ocean (or pool), rinse hair with the mineral water and comb through with a wide-tooth comb. It will take out both the chemicals and the tangles. An instant beat-the-heat trick is to squirt some water on the pulse points at the wrists, backs of the knees, and neck. And, finally, when the heat and the salt air start making you thirsty, take the top off the bottle and help yourself to a refreshing drink of water!

Moisturizer. I just can't say enough about the need to moisturize when you're out in the sun. Every time you come out of the water, reapply moisturizer to your skin. There are now moisturizers on the market that contain skin-protection factors.

Waterproof makeup bag. Makeup creams and pencils melt in the heat. The way to prevent this is by storing your makeup bag in a cooler. Heat is also a great medium for bacteria to flourish in. By keeping your cosmetics cool, you can prevent spoilage.

Lemons. Cut open a lemon and squeeze it on your hair. Done repeatedly at the beach, it will naturally streak your hair with the aid of the sun.

Foot cream. The sand on the beach acts as a natural pumice. Walk along the beach barefoot and the sand will polish away calluses and rough spots. Applying foot cream will further smooth your feet.

Makeup on the Beach

You have to decide what you want to *do* on the beach. If you're going to spend the day resting under an umbrella, with no intention of going near the water, then you can apply your makeup as you normally would. I suggest you do your makeup entirely with powders as the heat will cause creams to run.

However, if you're going swimming, or applying suntan lotion, makeup is obviously out of the question. If you think your eyes look naked without mascara, you might want to use a waterproof mascara. Personally, as I said earlier, I do not recommend waterproof mascaras as they tend to make eyelashes clump together. An alternative is to have your eyelashes dyed. The dye should last approximately six weeks and will eliminate the need for mascara. You must, however, have this done by a professional, licensed cosmetologist at a professional beauty salon.

Darker skin can carry more vibrant hues. Your summer makeup wardrobe can include deeper eye shadows, blushers, and lipsticks. For evening, pearlescents and powders shot with gold and bronze hues look exceptionally dramatic on golden skin.

Being beautiful while acquiring a tan is basically a matter of good sense. *Moderation* is the key word. And the earlier you start taking care of yourself when in the sun, the better your chances for young-looking skin as you mature.

13. Twenty Vital Do's and Dont's of Makeup

The wonderful thing about makeup is that it allows so much room for individuality and experimentation. While there are certain rules, there is still plenty of room for unique expression. However, there are certain principles that are not as flexible. Throughout the book, I have given you all the information you need to apply your makeup like a professional. In this chapter, I will reiterate twenty *vital* do's and dont's of makeup, because I believe that these points are crucial to doing your makeup like a professional. Next to each statement is the chapter that explains the point in greater detail.

1. **Do** moisturize your face and neck with moisturizing cream *every time* you put on makeup. (chapter 2)
   Don't put on makeup without a base of moisturizer or your makeup will streak, cake, and turn orange. (chapter 2)

2. **Do** apply foundation to the face with the fingers and blend well with a sponge wedge. (chapter 2)
   Don't use cotton to blend foundation. Stray cotton will stick to the face. **Don't** blend foundation with the fingers, either—you will not get a sheer coverage. (chapter 2)

3. **Do** remember to apply foundation to the entire face (including the lips, eyelids, and the front of the ears (and continue down on the neck). (chapter 2)
   Don't stop foundation at the chinline. You will be left with a telltale line where the foundation ends and your natural coloring begins, giving your face a masklike appearance. (chapter 2)

4. **Do** blend contour and highlight makeup correctly. Only a shadow should remain where the contour is applied. (chapter 2)
   Don't leave dark contour cosmetics on your face without blending properly. It will look like dirt on your face! (chapter 2)

5. **Do** apply multishades of eyeshadow to the upper eyelid. Do highlight the brow bone with a light-highlight eye shadow. (chapter 4)
   Don't use one shade of eye shadow and apply it over the entire upper eyelid and brow bone. One shade is not sufficient to show off the concave and convex areas of the eyelid. Avoid dark shadows on the brow bone. (chapter 4)

6. ***Do*** use two blushers—a light blusher for the cheekbones and a darker blusher that will act as a contour when applied in the hollow of the cheekbones. (chapter 3)

 Don't put dark blusher directly on the cheekbone. Light blusher should not fall below the cheekbone. (chapter 3)

7. ***Do*** apply eyeliner in a thin line as close as possible to the eyelashes. Soften the line by smudging with a sponge-tipped applicator or eyeliner brush. (chapter 4)

 Don't use a thick, dark line when lining the upper lid. It will look hard, harsh, and artificial. (chapter 4)

8. ***Do*** use a light blue pencil on the platform of the lower lid to make the eyes appear larger and the whites of the eyes appear whiter. (chapter 2)

 Don't apply dark colors to the platform of the lower lid. It will make the eyes appear smaller. (chapter 2)

9. ***Do*** remove the excess glob of mascara that forms at the end of the mascara wand. It causes the mascara to smear and clump on your lashes. (chapter 4)

 Don't hold the mascara wand horizontally. To coat each lash and make every lash count, hold the wand upright and work back and forth across the lashes. (chapter 4)

10. ***Do*** separate the lashes by combing them with an eyebrow brush or comb each time you apply a coat of mascara. (chapter 4)

 Don't apply too many coats of mascara or the lashes will clump together. Two coats applied properly will give the lashes the length, thickness, and darkness desired. (chapter 4)

11. ***Do*** keep eyebrows properly trimmed and shaped by proper tweezing. (chapter 5)

 Don't overtweeze brows. Years of excess tweezing can leave you with sparse brows that will not grow back. (chapter 5)

12. ***Do*** use an ice cube to freeze and anesthetize the eyebrow area before tweezing. (chapter 5)

 Don't tweeze eyebrows the night you are going out to a party. Some swelling or puffiness may occur. Instead, tweeze the night before. (chapter 5)

13. ***Do*** lighten or darken your brows by applying a brown eye shadow with an eyebrow brush. If you need to create brows that are missing, use a nylon-tipped eyebrow brush and, with feathery strokes, create brows using the proper shade of eye shadow. (chapter 5)

 Don't draw on missing brows with a grease eyebrow pencil. The effect is harsh and totally unnatural. (chapter 5)

14. ***Do*** outline the lips with a lip pencil. The extra wax in the pencil will keep lipstick from "bleeding." (chapter 6)

 Don't start your lining outside the natural lipline. (chapter 6)

15. ***Do*** fill in with a corresponding shade of lipstick. Use a sable lip brush for clean, definitive lines. (chapter 6)

 Don't use contrasting lipliner and lipstick. Lipliner and lipstick may be of slightly different shades, but the effect should not be obvious. Do not apply lipstick directly from the stick. You will not have the control necessary for sharp, even color. (chapter 6)

16. ***Do*** set your makeup with translucent powder for daytime and translucent iridescent powder for nighttime. (chapter 7)
    Don't forget to remove excess powder by buffing well with a large powder brush. (chapter 7)

17. ***Do*** remove every bit of makeup before you go to bed at night. Use cleansing cream, which will lubricate the skin as it removes makeup. (chapter 2)
    Don't remove makeup with a tissue. The tissue contains wood fibers that may irritate your face. (chapter 2)

18. ***Do*** pay particular attention to the makeup around the eyes. Remove hard-to-take off mascara with cotton balls dipped in mineral oil, or use prepared eye-makeup-remover pads. (chapter 3)
    Don't ever rub the area around the eyes when removing eye makeup. Gently pat with the makeup remover around the supersensitive eye area. (chapter 2)

19. ***Do*** always keep brushes and tools clean. Clean brushes by dipping them in rubbing alcohol and allowing them to dry naturally. (chapter 1)
    Don't lend or borrow cosmetics. This is especially true of eye makeup. Less-than-clean cosmetics and tools are a leading cause of eye infections. (chapter 1)

20. ***Do*** practice applying your makeup over and over again. Experiment with different looks. Practice makes perfect. (chapter 8)
    Don't wait for an important occasion to try a new makeup look. Your first attempt may be disappointing! (chapter 8)

Read and practice these instructions repeatedly until they become second nature to you.

14. The Fifteen Most Often Asked Questions About Makeup

In over twenty-five years as a makeup artist, I've heard almost every question *imaginable* about makeup and beauty. But during the hundreds of training seminars I've given and thousands of personal appearances I've made, the same questions keep coming up. And they come from women whose ages range from sixteen to sixty.

Since so many women I meet ask the same questions, I thought you might be wondering about similar problems. Here are the questions most frequently asked of the professional makeup artist (and the answers).

Q. How should a woman with glasses do her makeup?

A. A woman who wears glasses should do her makeup the same way as a woman who does not wear glasses, taking into account her eye shape, face structure, etc. The only time glasses are a consideration in makeup is when the glasses have magnified lenses—generally for people who are farsighted. Then you will want to use less makeup as the color will also be magnified. What is important for women who wear glasses is to choose the proper frames to go with their face shape—as described in chapter 12.

Q. How can you cover dark circles under the eyes?
What can you do about bags under the eyes?

A. Circles under the eyes can be hidden with a cream concealer. If the circles are very dark, use the concealer after you have applied moisturizer to the face, but before you have put your foundation on. After the foundation has been applied, cover the area under the eye with concealer again. Do not rub when applying concealer; instead, gently pat it on. If you have actual *bags* (puffy swelling) under the eyes, it is very difficult to cover with makeup. You've probably heard that these bags occur when you do not get enough rest. Unfortunately, this is a fallacy and it takes more than a good night's sleep to rid yourself of the problem. Most of the time, bags under the eyes are a problem of heredity, and often the only cure is plastic surgery. The bags under the eyes are actually deposits of fatty tissue, and once they are removed surgically, they generally do not recur. Since this problem is evident at an early age, I recommend that the surgery be done at an early age. If you are contemplating surgery, make sure you check carefully within your community to find a reliable and reputable plastic surgeon. I would suggest that you speak with and look at patients who have undergone the procedure so that you will know what to expect.

Q. How do I prevent my dark lips from showing through the lipstick?
A. Many women have a very dark pigment to their lips. It seems that no matter what shade of lipstick they use, the dark pigment comes through, completely changing the color of the lipstick. My recommendation is to put an extra coat of foundation base on the lips and blend lightly, leaving a thin coat on the lips; then apply lipliner and lipstick over the coat of foundation. This will generally work. If the pigment is *still* showing through, try a light coat of face powder over the foundation on the lips before applying lipstick.

Q. How do I prevent my mascara from smearing?
A. Mascara usually smears on the top of the eyelid, under the lower lashes, etc., because excess mascara is being applied. In automatic-wand mascara—the kind used by most women—the culprit is the glob of mascara usually found on the tip of the brush. If this excess is removed with a tissue, you will have better control and lashes will not smear or clump together. Use an eyebrow brush or comb that will separate lashes, remove the excess, and prevent it from smearing on the face. Another tip: When you are applying mascara, powder the lashes with translucent powder and give the lashes another coat of mascara, repeating each and every step.

Q. How do I prevent eye shadow from getting caught *in the crease of the eyelid?*
A. To prevent eye shadow from getting caught in the crease of the eye, make sure you apply both moisturizer and foundation to the eye area before applying the eye makeup. This is a step that many women forget. It will help the eye makeup cling to the eye area.

Using brushes to properly blend the makeup will prevent powder from becoming cakey and greasy upon the eye, and a final dusting of translucent powder will help to *set* the makeup. This will generally prevent eye makeup from catching in the crease of the eyelid.

I find that one of the biggest causes of makeup ending up in the crease of the eye is the use of liquid and cream eye shadows. It is one of the main reasons I personally prefer using only powdered eye shadows.

Q. *How do I keep my makeup from rubbing off on my clothes—especially when I am wearing light-colored clothing?*

A. The key to preventing makeup from coming off on clothing (and incidentally the right way to apply makeup) is to be sure to blend makeup properly. When applying foundation, which I recommend you continue onto the neck, make sure you take the time to blend the foundation with a sponge to the point where there is a very sheer coverage. When putting translucent powder on with the powder brush, it is again important to take the time to *buff vigorously* with the powder brush. This will keep excess powder from falling onto your clothes.

Q. *What is the easiest way to take off eye makeup?*

A. Eye-makeup-remover pads are best suited for removing makeup around the eye area. The oil removes the makeup easily and even takes off difficult-to-remove mascara. Work gently in a circular motion to loosen the mascara. After removing most of the makeup, any excess can be removed with a water-soaked cotton pad.

You can make your own pads by soaking cotton pads in mineral oil. If you find that you are still waking up in the morning looking like a panda, it is because you didn't take the time to really get off all the mascara. If your mascara seems to be exceptionally difficult to remove, you might consider changing brands.

Q. *How do you prevent lipstick from bleeding into the cracks and corners of the mouth?*

A. The best way to prevent lipstick from going outside the lipline is to line lips with a lipliner. Lipliner pencils contain more paraffin (wax) than lipsticks and will not bleed into creases or cracks of the mouth. Bleeding lipstick is most often a problem of mature women.

After lining the lips, find a corresponding lipstick and fill in the lip color. When touching up lipstick, take care to stay within the frame of the lipliner, which should remain firm until makeup is removed.

Q. *How can I cover a scar or demarcation on my face?*

A. Scars, birthmarks, demarcations, etc., often cause women to feel self-conscious. Most women overcompensate, which generally calls *more* attention to the area. In many cases, the best bet is to put makeup on as you normally would, paying no attention to the scar.

What I recommend to achieve better coverage for scars, birthmarks, etc., is a thick cream foundation. A thick cream foundation, plus a covering of translucent powder, will generally do the trick.

Q. *How do I make my eyes look larger?*
A. One trick that works on all women regardless of eye color, skin color, or age is to line the platform of the lower lid with a blue pencil. The blue pencil makes the whites of the eyes appear whiter, which in turn makes the whole eye area seem larger.

Q. *What can I do for dry (or oily) skin?*
A. On dry skin, be sure to use a good emollient-based moisturizer. Choose a foundation with an oil base to combat the natural dryness of the skin. Finish the makeup with a translucent powder containing emollients.

For oily skin, choose a water-based moisturizer and a water-based foundation.

Most women have skin that is oily in some parts while dry in other areas. This combination skin means that if you are treating your entire face as if it were excessively dry, you may be giving too much oil to certain areas. Conversely, although you may think you have only oily skin, there are dry areas of the face that could be adversely affected if, for example, you are using a skin freshener with a high alcohol content.

Q. *What is the difference between a daytime and a nighttime makeup?*
A. The differences start with foundation. You should match your foundation to your natural skin tone for daytime, while you can go two shades darker for night. Oil-based foundations should be used during the day for a dewy look; and water-based foundations, which will provide a matte look, should be used at night.

During the day, stay away from iridescent pearls for the eyes, lips, and cheeks. Those vibrant, iridescent, gleaming colors are for the evening. Choose a translucent powder to set your makeup for day. For evening, finish your makeup with a translucent iridescent powder. Lip gloss should be light for the day, heavier in the evening.

It is important to note that in many cases what is daytime makeup for one woman may be a party face to another. Of course, a lot depends upon your own taste, but the general outline I've given above provides good guidelines if you are in doubt.

Q. *What happens if all or part of my eyebrows are missing?*
A. Because of style changes (this is especially true for more mature women), women have gone from pencil-thin eyebrows to fuller, more natural brows.

Some women who tweezed their eyebrows found that their brows did not grow back when the style changed.

Most women worsen the problem by drawing on the missing portion of their brows with a grease eyebrow pencil, which creates a very unattractive, harsh look. The way to create natural-looking brows is to use a nylon-tipped eyebrow brush with an eye-shadow color that corresponds to the hair color, making short, feathery strokes to create an eyebrow shape.

Q. *Should I use waterproof mascara when I go swimming?*

A. I personally don't ever suggest waterproof mascara. I think it has a very unnatural look. It is only mascara with extra paraffin (wax), and it has a tendency to clump the lashes together.

When you are swimming, I recommend you not wear any makeup. If it is very important to you to have dark lashes while swimming, you can have your eyelashes professionally dyed. (Please see chapter 5 for details about eyelash dying.)

Q. *How can I find the right foundation for my skin tone?*

A. There are three basic skin-tone types: (1) pink/ruddy; (2) olive/sallow; and (3) beige (which has a tendency to lean either toward beige/sallow or beige/ruddy). There are two tones of foundation: beige and pink. You choose the foundation that will compensate for and balance your natural skin tone. Therefore, women with ruddy complexions should choose a beige foundation to tone down the redness. Women with sallow complexions can lose their yellowness by opting for a pink foundation.

15. How to Look Like a Model

Many young women dream of being models. As they read the popular fashion magazines, they picture themselves as the cover girl—made up, coiffed, and coutured to perfection. For most young girls, the dream ends when they realize they are not tall enough, thin enough, or photogenic enough for the incredibly competitive field of modeling. However, even if you are not going to be a professional model, you can still look like the cover girls you envy if you incorporate some of the top models' secrets into *your* beauty routine.

To you, the model's life seems to be one of luxury, endless parties, perfect smiles, and pretty clothes. While there is no denying that there is a lot of glamour in a model's life, there is also a lot of hard work. The key word in the beauty routine of a professional model is *discipline!* Being beautiful day in and day out is a full-time job. When a binge on chocolate cake can mean losing a swimsuit assignment, you think twice about how much you love chocolate!

All the models I know and have worked with have their own tricks and tips for looking their best. I am constantly learning new beauty techniques from the beautiful women I work with. I've gathered what I consider the best of their secrets to share with you. They are all beauty routines that you can easily incorporate into your life-style.

Always think about your beauty needs. That means don't just read a newspaper or watch the evening news—use the time as beauty time, too! Put a facial mask on first and then tune in your favorite news broadcaster.

Turn a disadvantage into an asset! Nose not perfect? Mouth too large? Lots of models have less-than-perfect features, but it doesn't keep them off the cover of *Vogue!* That's because their own sense of style enables them to turn a flaw into a trademark. Think of some of the most famous movie stars. Sophia Loren's mouth is much too large to be called perfect, but can you think of a woman with a more sensuous mouth?

Never be caught without a quick-makeup-repair kit. Buy duplicates of your favorite cosmetics. Keep one set at home, one in your handbag, and one in the office or car. This way you never have an excuse for looking less than beautiful!

Go bargain hunting for beauty. Although most models pose with the most expensive cosmetics, fragrances, and other beauty products, their massive make-up collections contain everyday beauty products readily found in drugstores and dime stores. For example, petroleum jelly is a wonderful lubricant for the under-eye area. Some of the old brand-name creams and cleansers have been around for ages, are inexpensive, and are still the best on the market.

Models also know that ordinary foods have super beauty benefits. Take a raw egg and separate the white from the yolk. The white portion, applied to your face, acts as a skin-tightening facial; the yolk, when mixed with mayonnaise, acts as a conditioner for dry hair. The most inexpensive instant facial can be had by emptying a tray of ice cubes into a bowl of water. By dunking your face into the bowl, you close pores, give the skin a healthy glow, and come away feeling totally refreshed.

Recipe for great-looking hair. You may cook with olive oil, but top cover girls also know it's a super treatment for shiny-looking hair. And, getting back to having fun and giving yourself a beauty treatment . . . while at the beach, pour some olive oil on your hair. Comb it through with a wide-tooth comb, then just bask in the sun. Heat is the best way to apply a conditioning treatment to your hair. If you mix the olive oil with the yolk of an egg, you can create an instant protein conditioner for your hair.

Learn the tricks of versatility. A model may pose as a young ingenue in the morning, switch to a working woman for the afternoon, and then be all done up as a siren for the evening. Most women don't have to change their looks as easily as a chameleon, but the point is not to get stuck in one look. What works for the PTA meeting is a little low-key for a night on the town. Learn to match your makeup to the occasion.

Sometimes it hurts to be beautiful! Exercise is the key way models keep their super shapes—that and diets that reek of discipline. Some models have very structured exercise routines, such as daily trips to their local gyms. Others jog, swim, ride horseback, or play tennis. All agree that the best and most fun method of exercising is dancing. Dancing keeps you firm, toned, and feeling good. You can dance at a nightclub or in your own home. Just turn on the radio, or put on your favorite record, and dance away!

The best beauty aid—water! Mineral water in a spray bottle is a beauty aid found in the large tote bags of most working models. It has several practical uses. It can perk up a limp perm, or set your makeup in hot weather, when translucent powders tend to build up and clog the pores.

Think beautiful. That means learn to love your best features and not dwell on an aspect of your face or body that displeases you. When you look in the mirror, concentrate on your *beautiful* eyes, not on a nose that is too wide! Beauty begins in the head. Every model will tell you that the days they *feel* beautiful are the days the camera catches that beauty!

Let your face breathe. Take a break from makeup. Deep-cleanse your face either with a professional facial or with at-home beauty products. Then take a twenty-four-hour break from makeup, making sure you use plenty of moisturizer on your face.

Invest in a good makeup mirror. Choose one with several light settings. The models I spoke with never use a magnifying mirror when applying their makeup. The magnification tends to distort the face and you won't get a true scale picture of your features.

Use, don't abuse, the sun. Most models can't afford to bronze their bodies, as a fashion shot might call for a winter look. Also, they know the damage the sun will do to your skin—especially the skin on your face. When you go out in the sun, make sure to use a good sun block, one with a high skin-protection factor. Tanning gradually and lightly will give you a honeylike glow and avoid the leather look.

You are what you eat. Every model knows that what you eat shows up on your face. Fried foods play havoc with complexion and hair. Most models live on simple foods, broiled, never fried, accompanied by fresh vegetables, with mineral water as their beverage. Sound boring? It is! But when your living is made from a beautiful face, the cheeseburgers get sacrificed.

You needn't be quite as strict with yourself, but when you think your face and hair need revitalizing, take a look at your diet and cut out the junk food.

Get it done professionally. *Every* model I spoke with insisted that if you color your hair, it must be done by a professional. At-home coloring is not even in a model's vocabulary, and it should be stricken from yours, too! Healthy, natural-looking color is one of your biggest beauty assets, and the expense is worth it.

Experiment with your cosmetics. Maybe the right shade of foundation for your skin color doesn't exist at the cosmetic counter. If so, do what models and makeup artists do—blend two or more shades together until the perfect tone is achieved. The same thing goes for lipstick. To tone down a too-bright shade, apply a darker foundation or darker lip color to the lips and then apply the brighter lipstick. You can lighten a too-dark shade of lipstick by applying a white pearl eye shadow to your lips after the lip color is on. Also, think of cosmetics as versatile products. A rose eye shadow can double as a blush; a copper eye shadow applied to the lips and covered with clear lip gloss becomes a fabulous evening lipstick!

These are just some of the tricks and tips of professional models. Everything you have learned about makeup in this book is the way top models are made up by makeup artists. You can learn more by reading the popular fashion magazines. Many issues share secrets of the models, and they are well worth reading.

As I've said throughout this book, it's the little things that make the difference between a plain makeup and a professional-looking makeup. The same is true of the outstanding beauty of professional models. While they are naturally attractive, it is the extra time and care they devote to their faces and bodies that turn them into head-turning beauties. By following some of their secrets, I'm sure you'll be turning a few heads yourself!

16. How to Become a Professional Makeup Artist

Many women I meet want to know how they can become makeup artists. Indeed, young girls who dream of becoming models, when asked what other career they might choose, often answer "Makeup artist."

It would be so easy if I could recommend schools that specialize in training men and women to become makeup artists. Unfortunately, few such schools exist, which makes it hard to learn the profession of makeup artist in the traditional education system.

The fact that these schools do not exist is an enigma to me. In many states, the law requires a professional cosmetologist's license before you can touch a woman's face. In order to receive that license, 1,000 hours must be spent practicing the trade. Of those 1,000 hours, practically none are spent learning how to become a professional makeup artist. Every hairdresser licensed to work in a beauty salon has a cosmetologist's license. The beauty schools concentrate on hair, not makeup. Since traditional classroom methods of study are not available, how do you go about becoming a professional makeup artist?

My recommendation is that you attend every available seminar given by professional makeup artists at the local professional trade shows. Call up the major convention centers in your area to find out when such shows are scheduled. These shows are invaluable because they are professionally oriented.

Cosmetic companies often send professional makeup artists to department stores to give beauty seminars. Most of these seminars are advertised in local newspapers. To plan your schedule in advance, call or write the promotion departments of the major cosmetic companies to find out when and where they will be holding educational programs.

You should also read every beauty book you can get your hands on, and subscribe to all the beauty magazines. Go to the library and look through old beauty magazines to see how makeup styles have changed. Don't neglect the foreign beauty magazines. Our European neighbors are often ahead of us in makeup and fashion trends.

Think of the beauty magazines as your textbooks. Study each photograph carefully, being fully aware that it was a *professional* makeup artist who made up the model. Look at the face feature by feature and notice how the makeup artist did the contouring and highlighting, the blush, lips, eyes, etc.

Begin to assemble the tools and cosmetics of a professional makeup artist. You will need *all* the tools and brushes described in chapter 1. You will also need a full range of colors for foundation, blushers, eye shadows, and lipsticks so that you have the right makeup colors for any woman you make up.

With all the data you accumulate and workshops you attend, the final step to becoming a professional makeup artist is practice, practice, practice! Constantly *doing* makeups will help you evolve into a professional makeup artist.

Finding subjects to practice on should not be any problem at all. Women *love* having their faces made up and you will find that your friends will let you practice on them over and over again. When you are experimenting on your friends' faces, try out the ideas you have learned from seminars, books, and magazines. If an idea works, incorporate it into your own point of view. If it isn't a viable idea, abandon it. The only way to become a good, professional makeup artist is through experimentation, trial and error, practice, and repetition.

It is the responsibility of the makeup artist to understand that makeup is fashion. Fashion is in a constant state of evolution and change. Fashion is what the eye becomes accustomed to. What may seem outrageous now could very well become fashionable five years from now. As a professional makeup artist, you have an obligation to keep abreast of fashion trends. Styles and color change with each season, and makeup is highly influenced by all of these changes.

To become a truly professional makeup artist, you must develop a sixth sense about women. Start with the understanding that each woman has an image of herself. She will expend a tremendous amount of energy both projecting and protecting that self-image. If a woman comes to you for a makeup consultation, understand that she may want a new look—but she is not looking for a new self-image. For example, if a woman perceives herself as a conservative type and you make her up like a show girl, she will not be happy with the results.

What the professional makeup artist must be able to do is *know*, just by looking at a woman's hair, clothes, and general presence, how she perceives herself and make her up accordingly. It's not easy at first, but the more women you see, the easier the process becomes. Always remember that women are coming to you, the professional, to be shown how to wear makeup. They are coming to you for help. You should be authoritative. Don't ask a woman which colors she likes to use. Instead, show her which shades and techniques are best for her.

My career has been based not just on making up women, but also on teaching them how to do it themselves. I believe it is the responsibility of every makeup artist to be a teacher, also. A woman should learn something from the experience of being made up by a professional.

After studying, learning, and practicing the art of makeup, I would suggest you offer your services as an apprentice to a makeup artist you respect and feel that you can learn from. As your work improves, it is a good idea to have a professional photographer take photos of your work so that you can begin to compile a portfolio. You will need a portfolio to show samples of your skill as a makeup artist when auditioning for job assignments.

If you develop the skills of a professional makeup artist, there are many exciting job opportunities within the profession. Some avenues to explore are:

Cosmetic companies. Many of the large companies hire makeup artists for personal appearances and promotions in stores throughout the country.

Photographic work. The beauty and fashion magazines have work for makeup artists for their editorial and advertising pages. Store catalogs are also a good avenue for investigation.

Theater companies. These always employ makeup artists. *Theater* does not mean just Broadway. There are touring and stock companies throughout the world.

Television and motion pictures. Makeup is *not* just for leading ladies! Even the anchor on the evening news receives makeup before she/he faces the cameras.

For theatrical makeup positions (stage, screen, and television), professional makeup artists must usually belong to the local guild or union. Find out what the requirements are for membership.

If your dream is to become a professional makeup artist, by following the course I've described, you can turn that dream into reality. The cosmetic industry in the United States alone is a multibillion-dollar-a-year business. There is tremendous opportunity for people who would like to embark on an exciting and glamorous career as professional makeup artists.

Index